Prenatal Diagnosis
The human side

Edited by
Lenore Abramsky
Genetic Counsellor, Queen Charlotte's and Chelsea Hospital,
London, UK

and

Jean Chapple
Consultant in Obstetric and Perinatal Epidemiology, North West
Thames Regional Health Authority, London, UK

CHAPMAN & HALL

London · Glasgow · Weinheim · New York · Tokyo · Melbourne · Madras

Published by Chapman & Hall, 2-6 Boundary Row, London SE1 8HN, UK

Chapman & Hall, 2-6 Boundary Row, London SE1 8HN, UK

Blackie Academic & Professional, Wester Cleddens Road, Bishopbriggs, Glasgow G64 2NZ, UK

Chapman & Hall GmbH, Pappelallee 3, 69469 Weinheim, Germany

Chapman & Hall USA, One Penn Plaza, 41st Floor, New York, NY10119, USA

Chapman & Hall Japan, ITP-Japan, Kyowa Building, 3F, 2-2-1 Hirakawacho, Chiyoda-ku, Tokyo 102, Japan

Chapman & Hall Australia, Thomas Nelson Australia, 102 Dodds Street, South Melbourne, Victoria 3205, Australia

Chapman & Hall India, R. Seshadri, 32 Second Main Road, CIT East, Madras 600 035, India

Distributed in the USA and Canada by Singular Publishing Group Inc., 4284 41st Street, San Diego, California 92105

First edition 1994

© 1994 Chapman & Hall

Photoset in 10/12pt Palatino by Intype, London
Printed in Great Britain by St Edmundsbury Press, Bury St Edmunds, Suffolk

ISBN 0 412 55360 0

A catalogue record for this book is available from the British Library

Library of Congress Catalog Card Number: 94-70264

∞ Printed on permanent acid-free text paper, manufactured in accordance with ANSI/NISO Z39.48-1992 and ANSI/NISO Z39.48-1984 (Permanence of Paper).

Prenatal Diagnosis

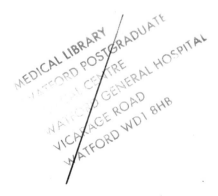

Contents

Contributors   vii
Preface   ix
Acknowledgements   xi

1   Ethical issues in prenatal diagnosis   1
    Susan Bewley

2   Legal issues in prenatal diagnosis   23
    Jonathan Montgomery

3   Women's experiences of prenatal screening and
    diagnosis   37
    Josephine M. Green

4   Screening issues – the public health aspect   54
    Jean Chapple

5   Counselling prior to prenatal testing   70
    Lenore Abramsky

6   Difficult decisions in prenatal diagnosis   86
    Christine Garrett and Lyn Carlton

7   The sonographer's dilemma   106
    Jean Hollingsworth

8   Preimplantation diagnosis   116
    H. Glenn Atkinson and Alan Handyside

9   Problems surrounding late prenatal diagnosis   134
    Lucy Turner

10 Problems surrounding selective fetocide   149
    Elizabeth M. Bryan

11 The parents' reactions to termination of pregnancy
    for fetal abnormality: from a mother's point of view   157
    Helen Statham

12 The parents' reactions to termination of pregnancy
    for fetal abnormality: from a father's point of view   173
    Ray D. Hall

13 Looking in from the outside   181
    Margaretha White-van Mourik

14 Caring for the carers   202
    Elizabeth Friedrich

Glossary   213
Useful addresses in the United Kingdom   222
Index   224

Contributors

Lenore Abramsky
Genetic counsellor, Queen Charlotte's and Chelsea Hospital, London, UK

H. Glenn Atkinson
Honorary Senior Registrar, Institute of Obstetrics and Gynaecology, Royal Postgraduate Medical School, Hammersmith Hospital, London, UK

Susan Bewley
Senior Registrar/ Subspeciality Trainee in Fetal Medicine, Fetal Medicine Unit, University College Hospital, London, UK

Elizabeth M. Bryan
Medical Director, Multiple Births Foundation, Queen Charlotte's and Chelsea Hospital, London, UK

Lyn Carlton
Specialist Health Visitor in Genetics, Kennedy Galton Centre, Northwick Park Hospital, Harrow, Middlesex, UK

Jean Chapple
Consultant in Public Health Medicine, North West Thames Regional Health Authority and Honorary Senior Lecturer, St Mary's Hospital Medical School, London, UK

Elizabeth Friedrich
Head of Staff Counselling, Hammersmith and Queen Charlotte's Special Health Authority, London, UK

Christine Garrett
Consultant in Clinical Genetics, Kennedy Galton Centre, Northwick Park Hospital, Harrow, Middlesex, UK

Josephine M. Green
Senior Research Associate, Centre for Family Research, University of Cambridge, Cambridge, UK

Ray D. Hall
Member of Support Around Termination For Abnormality

Alan Handyside
Senior Lecturer, Institute of Obstetrics and Gynaecology, Royal Postgraduate Medical School, Hammersmith Hospital, London, UK

Jean Hollingsworth
Superintendent Ultrasonographer, Hammersmith and Queen Charlotte's Special Health Authority, London, UK

Jonathan Montgomery
Lecturer in Law, University of Southampton, Southampton, UK

Helen Statham
Chair of Support Around Termination for Abnormality and Research Associate, Centre for Family Research, University of Cambridge

Lucy Turner
Sister, Fetal Medicine Unit, Queen Charlotte's and Chelsea Hospital, London, UK

Margaretha White-van Mourik
Genetic Counsellor and Research Fellow in Genetics, Duncan Guthrie Institute of Medical Genetics, Glasgow, UK

Preface

This book evolved out of a conference which was held because of our conviction that prenatal screening and diagnostic techniques provide carers with a two-edged sword which can do both good and harm – often at the same time to the same person.

The conference ('The Human Side of Prenatal Diagnosis') dealt with emotional, ethical and legal issues in prenatal screening and diagnosis. It took place in March 1992 at the Institute of Obstetrics and Gynaecology in London and was attended by obstetricians, paediatricians, geneticists, midwives and ultrasonographers from the North West Thames Health Region. The demand for places at the conference far exceeded the number of places available and many people who attended expressed the hope that we would be organizing similar conferences in the future. This confirmed our belief that we were not the only ones preoccupied with the human issues raised by the new technologies and encouraged us to work towards this publication.

Prenatal diagnosis and the possibility of selective termination of affected pregnancies is part of a wider move towards reproductive choice. Like contraception and assisted conception, it can make a major difference to the lives of some people. In our culture, we tend to view choice as a good thing. We look upon it as our right to choose our occupation, our partner, the place where we live, the books that we read and the way that we vote. However, we can point to other cultures in which these choices are not allowed and are not thought to be desirable. The whole idea of reproductive choice is bound by culture. Those of us working in maternity services would do well to keep this in mind.

Those who do believe that reproductive choice in the form of contraception is good may still feel that termination of pregnancy is unacceptable. Even those who feel that termination of pregnancy is acceptable will find that the termination of a wanted pregnancy is emotionally traumatic. What about the very many women who are pregnant with normal, healthy babies and who are made anxious by screening and diagnostic tests? What about women who lose healthy babies due to prenatal diagnostic tests? These are some of the costs of prenatal diagnosis.

We could of course make a very long list of the benefits of prenatal diagnosis, such as not having to suffer with a baby who is dying from Tay–Sachs disease or to receive the agonizing news that a much wanted newborn baby has Down syndrome.

We do not want to present arguments for or against carrying out prenatal diagnosis. The technology is here and will continue to grow. We want to inspire people to think about the consequences of all the tests being offered. We want them to consider how they can maximize the benefits of those tests while minimizing any harm. We want people to ask themselves why they are offering particular tests and whether they are doing it in the best possible way. We want them to reconsider how test results are passed on to women and their families and to think about whether follow-up support is adequate for couples and for staff.

All the contributors to this volume live and work in the United Kingdom, so the laws, practices and organizations cited are British. However, the issues are the same in any land and any culture in which prenatal screening and diagnosis is practised. The methods of dealing with the problems raised will differ over time and between cultures, but the problems themselves will be as constant as life and death, joy and sorrow. This book is also based on hospital practice, as this is where most diagnostic tests take place, but the issues are just as relevant for health workers in primary care.

In short, the aim of this book is not to pass on a large body of information; it is to make people think about issues that are vital to the emotional health of pregnant women, their partners and families, workers in the maternity services and society as a whole.

Lenore Abramsky
Jean Chapple
London, 1993

Acknowledgements

The human side of editing Prenatal Diagnosis: The human side

It is our own children who taught us the joy and problems of parenthood and helped us to understand the strong urge that people have to be parents of healthy children. It is to them – Sasha, Kolya and Tanya Abramsky and Jamie and Nicholas Chapple – that we dedicate this book. We also owe enormous gratitude to Jack Abramsky and Syd Chapple for accepting the disruptions caused to family life during the preparation of this book and for having enough confidence in us to provide continuous reassurance that one day it would all be over and we would get it to the publishers.

We greatly appreciate the good humour with which our chapter authors accepted our badgering (sometimes to the point of harassment) for their completed chapters. All of the authors put a great deal of time and effort into providing excellent contributions within the time scale requested. We would also like to thank our many colleagues who discussed these issues with us, helping us to clarify our ideas and suggesting sources of information and expertise. Other colleagues helped with the operational side of transferring ideas on to computer disc and thence to paper.

Finally, we would not even have conceived the idea of this book were it not for the thousands of couples who have generously shared with us their feelings, thoughts and fears – giving us some insight into the emotional processes activated by the various stages of prenatal diagnosis, from the mere thought of considering screening to dealing with the consequences of a termination of pregnancy because of fetal abnormality.

William Morris 1834–96

One of these cloths is heaven, and one is hell,
Now choose one cloth for ever; which they be,
I will not tell you, you must somehow tell
Of your own strength and mightiness.

Percy Bysshe Shelley 1792–1822

Alas! that all we loved of him should be,
But for our grief, as if it had not been,
And grief itself be mortal!

1

Ethical issues in prenatal diagnosis

Susan Bewley

DEFINITION OF PRENATAL DIAGNOSIS

Prenatal diagnosis is the identification of diseases of the fetus.

Prenatal diagnosis may be made non-invasively (by ultrasound for structural defects) or invasively (by a needling technique to obtain a sample of amniotic fluid, placenta or fetal blood). Invasive techniques carry a risk of fetal loss or damage.

Prenatal diagnosis can have three purposes:

- to inform and prepare parents for the birth of an affected infant;
- to allow *in utero* treatment or delivery at a specialist centre for immediate postnatal treatment;
- to allow termination of an affected fetus.

The present practice of prenatal diagnosis contains all three purposes, but termination currently dominates management. In most societies, diseases of neonates and children are considered afflictions, and many tolerate abortion. However, there is no consensus on this.

Why must we consider ethics?

Ethics has to be considered in relation to prenatal diagnosis:

- to decide whether an action is right or wrong;
- to guide us in the future when a similar situation occurs;
- for society to come to an agreed compromise about what is

and is not allowed. Law sets the limits of acceptable behaviour.

There may be a conflict between law and ethics. A particular action in a particular situation may be lawful but morally wrong, just as there can be right or good acts that are illegal. Some of the areas of ethical concern in prenatal diagnosis are introduced below.

ETHICAL ISSUES IN PRENATAL DIAGNOSIS

'Rights' of the fetus

What is the moral status of the embryo, fetus or newborn? Is there a difference between diagnosing cystic fibrosis in a pre-implantation embryo and diagnosing it at 10 weeks gestation? Do the unborn, who have no voice, have rights, to be protected in any way? Is there a right to live, whatever disease a fetus has? Some argue that fetuses cannot have rights, at least until they are born and individuals. If that were so, would there be no moral difference between kicking a pregnant and a non-pregnant woman in the abdomen?

When is abortion permissible?

Is abortion for congenital abnormality permissible? If so, why? If abortion is tolerated, how serious does the abnormality have to be? What is the difference between aborting for spina bifida, thalassaemia, cleft lip, club foot, sex and eye colour? How late can it be performed? Is there a difference between abortion for Down syndrome discovered at 20 weeks or at birth? If abnormal fetuses can be killed, is euthanasia – the deliberate killing – of neonates, children or adults also acceptable? Should doctors be allowed to give lethal injections to infants with anencephaly or severe complications of prematurity, or to the brain-dead?

How much disability?

Does abortion of an abnormal fetus degrade or affect adults with the same disease? If the law makes a difference between a third trimester fetus with and without spina bifida and hydrocephalus (i.e. one can be killed and the other cannot), does that send a message to the disabled that they are worth less than the able-bodied? Is it wrong for parents to bring sick children into the world? Are parents who do not abort fetuses with chronic conditions that shorten life and cause suffering (such as beta thalassaemia) cruel? They could, after all, have an abortion and try again for a healthy child. If they do not wish to, should society pay the cost of their choice?

Are the risks acceptable?

Are there risks to the mother or fetus that are unacceptable? Some conditions, such as diaphragmatic hernia, can be operated on *in utero*. The fetus has to be removed from the womb for the operation. The mother requires several major operations and the fetus may be born prematurely. Increasingly, these treatments will move from the experimental to the clinical arena. Should there be limits to the risks taken?

Who is the patient?

Who is the patient/client? The mother, parents, family, future person or future society? If a family have genetic counselling and one member is gently pressurized into testing for linkage studies, is that the family's business? Should the counsellor take sides, see each person individually, or accept the consensus opinion? Is it different if the pressure is extremely strong, or if the family member is a child, or a 13-year-old, or mentally ill, or just weak-willed? Who decides whether to test or not? Is it the parent, the counsellor, the operator or a combination of all? If there is a disagreement about testing, whose view prevails? If an explicit request is made for sex selection so that a firstborn male can inherit a title, who says yes or no? What if a mother refuses life-saving treatment for her fetus? If the fetus will die or be damaged if a woman does not agree to treatment, such as a transfusion for Rhesus disease, or a caesarean section for fetal distress, should she be forced to help her fetus, or be punished? If not, why not, as the same refusal after birth can be overruled?

The effects on family relationships

Are conflicts of interest inevitable? Can looking after the genetic health of a family oppress individuals? Does prenatal diagnosis affect parent–child relationships? Can we show an improvement when the mother is reassured and the child is really wanted? Does choosing the quality of a fetus make it a consumer object? As more and more genetic tendencies are elucidated, why not choose a fetus that is unlikely to get hypertension and diabetes in later life, and who will be guaranteed to be handsome, athletic and ambitious? Does screening of the general pregnant population increase maternal anxiety? Do ultrasound and serum screening (alpha fetoprotein and Down risk) make women obsessed about certain diseases out of proportion to the range of potential problems? Should there be different rules for the risk/benefit ratio in offering prenatal diagnosis to low risk and high risk populations?

Confidentiality and ownership of information

When can or should confidentiality be broken? If a person refuses to let siblings know that they are at risk of carrying abnormal genes, such as fragile X, and these could be passed on to innocent, as yet unconceived, fetuses, should we not break confidentiality to prevent harm? Why protect people who are so unconcerned for their family members? What if the putative father is not the genetic father? Does the man have a right to know that the fetus is not his, if this is discovered during the course of prenatal diagnosis? Who owns genetic information? If genetic information is common amongst family members, do they not have an interest or even right to know each other's results?

This list is not exhaustive, and new technologies will continue to pose more dilemmas. There are no easy, definitive answers to the questions. Arguments about the moral status of the fetus, the permissibility of abortion and the nature of the doctor–patient relationship (or genetic professional and client) lie at the heart of many of the ethical issues in prenatal diagnosis. The aim of this chapter is to analyse ethical disagreements, with particular reference to prenatal diagnosis. Some theoretical concepts will be explained and then practical suggestions will be made for dealing with conflicts.

PHILOSOPHICAL ETHICS

Approaches

There are several approaches to ethics.

1. Descriptive

We can measure ethical beliefs at a certain time in a certain place. Some beliefs appear to be universal (murdering your neighbour is wrong) whilst others are not (abortion ranges from being considered murder to being regarded as a form of contraception). We may be able to measure what our present beliefs are, but this is not helpful in determining what they should be.

2. Intuitive

In a new situation we might react intuitively to decide whether something is right or wrong. Intuitions may be worth attention, in that they have evolved over the years and are quicker than thought processes, but they are not infallible. Overcoming 'gut reactions' is part of professional training.

3. Rational argument

Philosophers, lawyers and politicians are experts in arguing (but are not always rational!). Philosophers practise the skills and test the logic of arguments. They do not all agree, so we do not have to automatically accept what they say.

If intuitions come into conflict with rational argument, then one must give way. Either the intuition is suppressed or dogged irrationality prevails, and each is potentially hazardous. Alternatively, the discrepancy can be examined in detail to find the flaw in the intuition or the arguments.

The tools

Philosophers use various tools to examine arguments:

- analysis of words and issues;
- drawing of distinctions;
- using logic;
- trying thought experiments to test theory.

Philosophers point out that two people may be using the same word in a different sense and mistakenly think they are talking about the same thing. Being precise about the definitions of words clarifies much conflict. There may be different implications of terms such as 'rights' and 'responsibilities' (see Moral frameworks below). They may distinguish two situations that appear superficially similar but are actually different, and show how the difference is morally relevant.

Although philosophers can be vexing when they use unreal examples ('What if a Martian requested prenatal diagnosis to abort on the basis of skin colour?'), the purpose of thought experiments is to test a theory or belief. This is similar to scientific experiments, where observations are made to confirm or refute hypotheses. Imagining an unreal situation frees us from everyday prejudices and allows logical thought. If the result of the thought experiment is uncomfortable or unacceptable, maybe there was something wrong with the original intuition or underlying theory.

The components of moral acts

The key to those actions that have ethical significance lies in the interplay of a moral agent performing an action on an object of moral significance. The action could be a prenatal diagnosis consultation, an abortion or a promise of confidentiality. The interplay is depicted in Figure 1.1.

Moral frameworks

There are three main theoretical moral frameworks that underpin discussions of morality. They can be envisaged as three viewpoints on any moral action, looking primarily at the actor, the object or the consequences of the act.

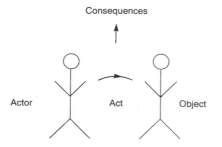

Consequences

Actor   Act   Object

Figure 1.1 The components of moral acts.

1. Duty-based (conscience and motives paramount)

This is, broadly speaking, the religious framework, although there are secular versions. It concerns itself with the motivation and intentions of the actor. It is God who will judge the contents of our hearts, although it may be individual conscience in a secular version. We have duties or obligations to others. Any rights they have stem secondarily from our duty. Thus, the 'right to life' only stems from the duty not to kill. This duty exists whatever the other person says about it, even if they have no voice. Rights in this morality thus do not have much force, although they are persuasive rhetorical devices.

2. Goal-based (morality objectively determined by outcome)

This is the consequentialist or utilitarian approach developed in the 19th century ('the greatest happiness for the greatest number'). Actions have consequences and outcomes. There is nothing inherently right or wrong in any particular action; it does not depend on the intention of the actor, it depends only on the outcome. Humans are motivated by pleasure, and increasing it is the purpose of morality. We should all be acting so as to maximize good outcomes.

A major criticism of utilitarianism is that one may be sacrificed for the good of many. Also, no-one has inherent value. It depends on qualities the person or thing possesses, such as sentience, the ability to feel pain or pleasure or make choices, intelligence, etc. (Indeed, it might be species prejudice to give more value to a human fetus than an adult monkey if it has more of the relevant qualities.)

3. Rights-based (rights providing protection)

This approach has largely developed from the political arena – 'All men are equal and have certain inalienable rights'. People have inherent rights. Duties towards them stem secondarily from their rights. This is a most powerful interpretation of rights. For example, if people have a right (to vote, or to be educated) that is not being fulfilled there is a strong claim on others to do something to rectify the situation. Such strong rights have certain characteristics: they can be waived (you do not have to use your vote); they can only be held by those capable of making autonomous choices (they are meaningless otherwise); and they trump other moral considerations. If a woman has this kind of right to prenatal diagnosis (stemming from some basic right to reproduction), doctors are obliged to carry it out.

Few people are total purists and the theories are being constantly modified and refined. In real life, features of all these moralities seem to coexist. There is an uncomfortable amalgam of parts of all. Maybe that is because we live in a pluralistic society, or because humans have incompatible parts to our characters or internal psychology. It is not possible to look from all directions at once. There is an underlying fundamental struggle between these philosophies. Each version is put forward as a total explanation for our everyday beliefs, and tries to incorporate its critics. Thus, when a new problem is analysed by each group, a different answer may emerge.

Illustration of the different moral theories

Let me try to illustrate the way the different fundamental approaches to a moral problem work: first, how taking the different viewpoints might explain the morality of an action; secondly, how changing one fact may change the rightness or wrongness of an action, but differently for each morality.

It is worth imagining that the theories are like different political parties trying to attract voters. Three philosophers representing each of the theories are trying to win your intellectual vote or allegiance. They all agree that murder is wrong, but for different reasons. I am going to use the example of killing an adult human for the time being so as not to confuse matters with the issue of abortion or prenatal diagnosis yet. I shall give their general explanations and then change one fact to show how the morality might change.

> Mr X stabbed the postman, who then died. Three philosophers agree that it was wrong and that Mr X should be punished. Why?

Philosopher 1 – duty

It was wrong because X had a duty not to harm or kill others. He formed an evil intention and carried it out, and is a wicked person for doing so. By contrast, if X made a genuine mistake, thinking the postman was a cardboard cut-out, not a person, then he would be blameless. The knife would have killed the postman, but X would not have murdered him, in that he had no intention of so doing. (The other two philosophers might still hold that it was wrong.)

Philosopher 2 – goal

It was wrong because people want to live and to carry out their plans and desires. The benchmark of moral value is the maximization of happiness or welfare. X may have enjoyed killing him but the postman suffered the loss of his life, his family are distraught and everyone in the neighbourhood is now terrorized. The world is a worse-off place for this murder, and therefore it was wrong. By contrast, if X killed Adolf Hitler as he was rising to power, and changed the course of history for the better, then it would have been a right action. Note that it would not be a wrong action that was justified, but actually right. (The other two philosophers would still hold that it was wrong.)

Philosopher 3 – right

It was wrong because the postman had a right to live that was inalienable. He was the only person who could waive this right. He did not agree or consent to being killed. X violated his right to live, and therefore committed a wrong. By contrast, if the postman had asked X to do it, having carefully considered and chosen death, there would be nothing wrong in the action. (The 'duty' philosopher would still hold that it was wrong. The 'goal' philosopher would determine whether, overall, the harms of allowing killing with consent outweighed the benefits of such a policy, before deciding whether it was right or wrong).

The three moral theories are summarized in Figure 1.2 and Table 1.1.

Table 1.1 Summary of moral frameworks

Theory	Duty	Goal	Right
History	Traditional	19th century	20th century
Central value	Inherent moral worth	Maximization of welfare	Autonomous choices
Key words	Duty, obligation, responsibility	Welfare, utility, happiness, usefulness	Right, choice, autonomy
Abortion	Usually wrong; might be right if 'lesser of two evils'	Right if mother's preference; might be obligatory if abnormality	Always right as mother's right to choose
Psychology	Superego	Id	Ego

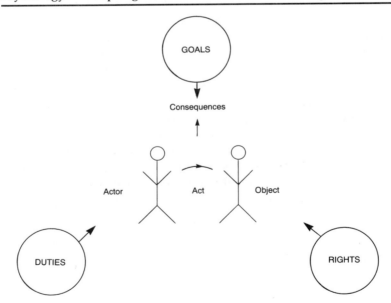

Figure 1.2 Summary of moral frameworks.

There are important theoretical battles being waged over the different theories of ethics. Although over simplified, these thumbnail sketches may help to untangle the arguments put forward for different aspects of prenatal diagnosis. The actual situation is much more complicated, as each theory contains elements of the others, and there are a range of views within the theories.

To return to prenatal diagnosis: if the knife is changed for a sampling needle or suction cannula and the postman for a fetus, how and why does the morality change? Firstly, do fetuses count at all? It is useful to consider what gives an object moral worth or status.

MORAL STATUS
Who has moral status or moral value?

Adult humans normally have full moral status whereas property, such as chairs, does not. People are protected by this: one cannot be harmed, killed or incarcerated without good reason, but there is nothing wrong in selling or burning an old chair. What is the morally relevant difference between a person and a chair?

What makes us important?

If we agree that people have moral status and chairs do not, does that help determine whether fetuses have moral status? The answer will depend on the qualities that are considered to be those which give adult humans moral value. What qualities give status? The answer could range from merely being human (in which case all humans from conception may have full moral status) to having the ability to make autonomous choices (in which case many humans, such as fetuses and children, may not have it). Or it may be something else or something in between. If it were usefulness or the ability to give pleasure to others, a Chippendale chair might have more value than fetuses and many humans.

Range of status

There may also be a range of status, from none to full. For instance, animals (generally) have some moral status. A horse can be bought and sold (like property), but we think it is wrong to throw one alive on a bonfire (unlike the chair) (Table 1.2).

Table 1.2 Range of moral status

Full moral status	Some moral status	No moral status
Adult humans	Animals	Property/plants

Where do other objects of moral value fit in the above table, and why? Do gametes, fetuses, children, incompetent adults, dying and dead humans have no, some or full moral status? Do adult humans all have equal full moral status, or do some (such as the brain-dead) have less than others?

There is a time before we exist (except as twinkles in our parents' eyes). How do we progress from non-existence to full status? Is it a sudden change at conception or birth? Or a gradual change with increasing development of the fetus and child? Do future, potential generations count; and if so why, and by how much?

Fetal moral status

There are three possibilities.

1. A fetus has full moral status. Its life cannot wantonly be put in danger (so invasive testing is not usually justified) and it has a right not to be killed (so abortion is wrong, indeed it is murder). This is an extreme deontological or duty-based view, corresponding to the Roman Catholic position.
2. A fetus has no moral status. In this case, it does not enter the moral arena at all (unless its parents wish to endow it with some sentimental protection). If a mother wishes to have a termination, no wrong is committed. This would be an extreme view. If a third trimester fetus had no status, why should a newborn have any? It would be very difficult to see why there should be anything wrong with infanticide (of normal or abnormal babies), apart from the effect on third parties.
3. The fetus has some moral status, but not as much as adults. Now a complex balancing act will have to be performed when there is a conflict of interests or rights. If a fetus has more

moral status as pregnancy progresses, then justification for abortion will have to become stronger with gestation. And it is possible that, while some abortions will be right, others will be wrong and unjustified killings (which may still not amount to murder, as they are killings of something less than an adult). Moderate deontologists (duty-based) would hold this view. Utilitarians tend to accord the fetus some status, but may do it through the eyes of the mother. If she wishes to have the fetus it is valued, but if not, then it is not. This is actually a view that gives the fetus no inherent worth, and would properly belong to (2) above. Utilitarians may also suggest viability as the time when the fetus can be treated as a patient, but again, this suggests that it has no inherent worth.

ABORTION

There are a wide variety of opinions about abortion, but they fall into several major camps; one argument derives from a maternal perspective and three from a fetal perspective.

Maternal argument – women's rights over their bodies

In this argument, the moral status of the fetus is irrelevant and abortion is justifiable as women have dominion over their own bodies. People believing this have to explain whether there are any abortions that would be wrong, such as terminations in the third trimester for very minor abnormalities.

Fetal arguments – full, no or some moral status

Full moral status

A person who believes in the absolute sanctity of life from conception, which can never be intentionally ended, must reject all abortions, even in cases of rape or fetal abnormality. It is a shame, but unavoidable, that parents will be caused suffering if abortion is always refused (e.g. families coping for a lifetime with an unwanted handicapped child or having to watch newborns die from such disorders as pulmonary hypoplasia or anencephaly).

No moral status

A person who believes that abortion is justifiable because the fetus is not a 'person' with rights will also have to accept termination for the most trivial reason and may need to explain whether there is any distinction between termination of pregnancy and infanticide.

Some moral status

Those who are left with the more pragmatic and pluralistic view that the fetus develops increasing moral status throughout pregnancy and that abortion must be explicitly justified as the lesser of two evils (killing a fetus versus harm to an adult human or her other children) have a view that corresponds to the law in most Western countries. If a pregnancy is unwanted because of abnormality this is considered justification enough.

Additional considerations for congenital abnormality

The moral status of the fetus is central to the acceptability of abortion when a mother has an unwanted pregnancy that affects her life, health or lifestyle. Prenatal diagnosis is often made in pregnancies that were wanted, but changed to unwanted when an abnormality was found. There are additional ethical dilemmas when considering termination of fetuses with congenital malformations.

- How severe does the malformation have to be for a termination to be justified?
- How late can diagnosis and termination be justified?
- Does the distinction between fetuses reflect into adult life?

These moral questions are not for parents and doctors alone to answer and society, through the revised United Kingdom Abortion Act, has recently created some new difficulties. There is now no upper time limit for termination if there is 'a substantial risk that if the child were born it would suffer from such physical or mental abnormalities as to be seriously handicapped'. Can an ethical justification be made by any of the camps for having a different gestation rule for abortion of the abnormal fetus? This new distinction between normal and abnormal fetuses might discriminate against the disabled amongst us. If a handicap *in utero* distinguishes fetuses who can be aborted and those who cannot, do adults with the same handicap also have less moral status and protection from being harmed? Differences in gestation limits between terminations for abnormality or social reasons might indicate changing values about adults, unless a special argument, to do with future suffering, can be made for late abortions.

SPECIAL RELATIONSHIPS

Let us next consider what governs the relationship between the health professional and the pregnant woman regarding prenatal diagnosis. The moral relationship of any two humans starts out as that which we would expect of two strangers (maybe there is not much of an obligation to help one another out, but each has a right not to be harmed by the other).

In addition to this basic relationship, there are a variety of special moral relationships including those between parent and child, teacher and pupil, shopkeeper and customer and between friends. These may entail greater obligations and rights than the relationship between two strangers. A parent is expected to make financial sacrifices to help his/her children, whereas a shopkeeper is not. A teacher is supposed to educate his/her pupils, whereas a friend is not. In prenatal diagnosis, the important special relationships are mother–fetus and doctor–patient. The professional might be a doctor, midwife or genetic counsellor, but the models described apply to all. I have tended to use the term 'patient' throughout (meaning a person attending a doctor for care), although 'client' or 'customer' have also been proposed. All are value-loaded terms implying different ethical camps before we even analyse what the relationship is! 'Parent' applies equally to mother and father, although only the woman is pregnant. 'Client' or 'customer' may imply a more contractual and less caring relationship than 'patient'.

Different versions of the doctor–patient relationship

There are two main versions of the doctor–patient relationship.

1. Traditional, beneficence (doing good) approach

The doctor must do his/her best for the patient to prolong life and relieve suffering. Need is assessed objectively by the professional and is not merely accepted as a subjective experience. This approach has been thought to lead to extreme paternalistic 'doctor knows best' behaviour and, although traditional, is being challenged. Paternalism may be modernized (by incorporating more respect for patient empowerment and choices into doing good) or rejected outright for another model.

2. Modern, autonomy (freedom to choose) approach

To replace the beneficence model, the relationship may be described as a professional–client relationship, where the passivity expected of patients is rejected. The professional must maximize life-enhancing potentials by restoring health and respecting autonomous choices. If an autonomous and informed client really wants a certain procedure, in the belief that it will enhance life, then the doctor is obliged to give it.

Both traditionalists and modernists, paternalists and utilitarians, claim that they wish to construct a more equal relationship between partners, and want to respect both beneficence and autonomy. However, when pushed, one of the central principles, beneficence or autonomy, must give way.

Basic components of the doctor–patient relationship

Some of the central components of the doctor–patient relationship and their description in different moralities are shown in Table 1.3. The reasons the qualities are central to the special relationship are subtly different depending on the viewpoint. Present professional guidelines are based on a duty-based view of the doctor–patient relationship.

Taking confidentiality as one example, there are profound implications. A promise of confidentiality given to a patient, from a duty-based viewpoint, should not be broken, as it is wrong to break promises unless a greater wrong is committed (such as allowing a patient to commit a serious crime). If respecting confidentiality is right-based, the information belonging to

Table 1.3 The components of the doctor–patient relationship

Quality	Duty	Right	Goal
Confidentiality	To keep promises	To have confidences kept	Useful to protect history and secrets
Consent	To respect bodily integrity	Not to be interfered with	Examination and investigations permitted
Competence	Doctor must do his/her best	To have a good doctor	Helpful to have high standard of management

and given by the patient should be absolutely protected (the only exceptions being when the patient agrees or is incompetent). If it is goal-based, the decision whether to respect or breach confidentiality would depend on the balance of harms and goods. Confidentiality is useful to encourage patients to give private information, but sometimes it would be right for doctors to breach confidentiality to give important information to others.

Who is the patient/client?

This may be each person at a time, the mother and father together, a whole family or the fetus. If more than one person at a time is the patient/client, then conflicts of interest may arise. Fetuses, siblings and parents may have different interests in the results of prenatal diagnosis, which they exert to effect on one another. If a doctor's job is to do the best for each individual, then treating couples or families as whole units means that sometimes one person's interest will be sacrificed for another's. There is no problem when the interests of the different parties coincide or overlap, but this is not always the case. Traditional doctor–patient relationships are based on a one to one promise of care. Genetic counselling has often taken a wider view of families and extended families.

Non-directive counselling and informed consent

These ideological tenets sound irreproachable. After all, who would recommend directive counselling or uninformed consent? Aside from the practical problem of achieving non-directiveness, what is the purpose or virtue of non-directive counselling? Are we aiming for non-directive counselling because it is the way to do the best for patients, or because it enhances their autonomous reproductive choices? This is not an irrelevant distinction, because in an extreme case where doing best and choice collide, the doctor will end up with different decisions. For example, if a woman requested a second chorionic villus sample and explained rationally, having had non-directive counselling, that she was particularly anxious and needed reassurance that a mistake had not been made in the laboratory, what should the doctor do? She fully understands the higher chance of miscarriage but says it is her body, her risk and her choice. A traditionalist doctor who sees non-directive counselling as a means of doing good, not an end in itself, might refuse to repeat the chorionic villus sample as it is harmful. A modernist doctor believes that non-directive counselling is an aim in itself, something that is necessary to enhance autonomous choices. This doctor then has two courses of action: either to do the repeat chorionic villus sample, as this is this woman's carefully considered personal choice, or to declare that she is too irrational and anxious to be autonomous, so the request does not have to be fulfilled.

A similar problem can occur with informed consent. How informed does it have to be? Do we give general details, enough information to make a decision or full information so that all the implications can be considered? What happens if the information is not understood in fine detail? Can too much information about prenatal diagnosis actually do harm by making people anxious or paralysed by indecision? Again, the question is whether information is a means to doing good (in which case the doctor may judge when enough has been given) or necessary in itself to achieve autonomy (in which case the patient decides, and articulate patients are entitled to as much time as they require).

Non-directive counselling and informed consent are often described as vital to avoid the manipulation of parents and suggestions that prenatal diagnosis and abortion are being used to improve the human race (reminiscent of Nazi eugenic policies to rid the world of diseased people). However, is there actually anything wrong with the aim of having less genetic disease and suffering in the world (rather than the means to achieve it)? And does non-directive counselling really protect against the charge of eugenics? Imagine that a gene for homosexuality was discovered and parents wanted, after very careful non-directive counselling, to abort homosexual fetuses, would that make it acceptable? Counsellors give the facts and allow people with beliefs about the value of different humans to act on them. Is that really morally neutral, or could it be eugenics by collusion or default? Does fulfilling non-directive counselling just let health workers off the moral hook while allowing parental prejudice full sway? It might be considered to be a private matter for parents since they have to bring up the children.

DEALING WITH CONFLICT

Many situations induce a feeling of ethical unease: 'I'm not sure that this is right. I feel very uncomfortable with this decision or course of action. I am being pressurized into something that feels wrong'. Such conflicts can be between professionals, between professionals and their individual patients or between professionals and society. There are often many layers to a problem. Some, such as communication problems, inexperienced staff or inadequate resources, may be resolvable. Fundamental ethical conflicts cannot be resolved, but may be clarified.

When an ethical problem arises in real practice, there are several ways to deal with it.

1. **Recognize the problem**. Ethical unease should be attended to. What is the dilemma? By talking about and analysing a problem, it can usually be broken down into its component parts, medical, social, psychological or ethical.
2. **Return to medical facts**. Good and accurate information about prognosis or the risk/benefit ratio of a course of action often settles ethical dilemmas, as they then prove to be less acute or contentious than at first sight. Whatever the moral framework, there is a strong obligation for professionals in the field to be well trained and updated. It is mistaken to guess, bluff or fail to ask for help when needed.

3. **Identify the different parties and the different interests**. It may be that someone has a very strong case, but it is nothing to do with professional obligations. Regular sympathy may be all that is required. Health professionals tend to want to help everyone, including future generations, but it is not clear that they have to do so.

4. **Examine personal feelings**. Sometimes the ethical unease is a personal sensitivity (related to personal experience of disease or fertility problems). Is a course of action being followed while ignorant or inexperienced? Fear of failure or stepping out of line can be powerful inhibitors of rational thought. Is there an emotional element whereby this particular patient evokes powerful feelings of concern, anger or helplessness? 'Know thyself' is important for getting out of self-made ethical dilemmas. By contrast, are some insights so uncomfortable or painful that they are being suppressed by strong beliefs (religious, political or ideological)?

5. **Are there pressures to cut ethical corners?** There may be financial pressures from a fee-paying patient or the salary-paying employer or career pressures to coerce patients to take part in research.

6. **Communication skills**. Many conflicts arise from poor communication or understanding of the patient's story, situation or experience. Breakdowns of communication may be avoidable and are often capable of remedy.

7. **Professional codes of conduct**. General guidance is given in the *General Medical Council Blue Book* (and its equivalents in other countries) and by the Royal Colleges of Nurses and Midwives. Specific guidance is sometimes offered from specialty organizations.

8. **Obtain a second opinion**. It is helpful to articulate a problem for clarification. Colleagues may help elucidate the key issues in a complex case, confirm the proposed course of action, or be prepared to take a different course of action.

9. **Obtain a legal opinion**. The law acts in a practical way to resolve disputes between parties in society. When ethical dilemmas are seemingly insoluble, an opinion from a medical defence society or medical lawyer may help.

10. **New law – from the courts and Parliament**. In the highly

contentious area of reproduction, and with new advances in technology, the law sometimes frames the limits of acceptable medical behaviour. Parliament may make limiting or enabling law as a reflection of public opinion.

11. **Continued ethical education**. This can be achieved by reading journals or books, attending courses and listening to patients and their concerns. Ethical case presentations can be brought to multidisciplinary groups for discussion. Everyone involved in prenatal diagnosis should be constantly reassessing their opinions and views, and be prepared to explain the ethical stance they take.

12. **Continuing debate in society**. A creative debate continues among and between professionals and the general public. This occurs through the media, professional journals, ethics groups and special interest groups. Toleration of different views and respect for the goodwill of opponents are qualities that help mutual understanding, if not agreement. Philosophers, theologians and lawyers may help untangle problems, although it is unlikely that there will ever be an ethical expert who can be called in to solve all the problems raised by prenatal diagnosis!

ACKNOWLEDGEMENTS

I would like to thank Dr Sophie Botros for helpful discussions about the analysis of medical ethics, and the Dunhill Medical Trust who supported my training as subspecialty trainee in fetal medicine.

FURTHER READING

Brock, D.J.H., Rodeck, C.H. and Ferguson-Smith, M.A. (eds) (1992) *Prenatal Diagnosis and Screening*. Churchill Livingstone, Edinburgh – Textbook about techniques, indications and diseases.

Cohen, M., Nagel, T. and Scanlon, T. (eds) (1974) *The Rights and Wrongs of Abortion*. Princeton University Press, Princeton, NJ – A Philosophy and Public Affairs reader, including the best account of women's right to choose abortion.

Gillon, R. (1986) *Philosophical Medical Ethics*. John Wiley & Sons, New York – Introduction to the four principles of biomedical ethics.

Glover, J. (1990) *Causing Death and Saving Lives*. Penguin, Harmondsworth – A well-written, utilitarian approach to medical ethics and other life and death moral issues.

Harris, J. (1989) *The Value of Life. An Introduction to Medical Ethics.* Routledge, London – A comprehensive guide to medical ethics based on the values of worthwhile lives of persons.

Kuhse, H. and Singer, P. (1987) *Should the Baby Live? The Problem of Handicapped Infants.* Oxford University Press, Oxford – An argument for euthanasia of handicapped infants.

Raphael, D.D. (1990) *Moral Philosophy.* Oxford University Press, Oxford – An excellent introduction to moral philosophy.

Sutton, A. (1991) *Prenatal Diagnosis: Confronting the Ethical Issues.* The Linacre Centre, London – A Catholic approach, against prenatal diagnosis for the purpose of selective abortion.

Wetherall, D. (1991) *The New Genetics and Clinical Practice, 3rd edn, Oxford University Press, Oxford – Basic textbook on genetics and the new advances in molecular biology.*

2

Legal issues in prenatal diagnosis

Jonathan Montgomery

INTRODUCTION

The law plays a number of functions in relation to health care practice. It structures the relationship between professionals and patients/clients, setting the ground rules on which the health professions practise. Thus the laws governing consent, access to health records and confidentiality help to determine the character of the therapeutic relationship, hopefully as a partnership rather than one dominated by either a paternalistic professional or a consumerist patient. The law also has a role in setting limits to acceptable practice on behalf of society. Controversial ethical issues, such as those which arise when the termination of pregnancy is being considered, are regulated through a legal framework. This will rarely force a single solution upon unwilling professionals and clients, but it will often rule out some options.

The law also has an important function as a mechanism for enforcing these basic principles. It provides remedies to enable patients/clients to vindicate their rights. Sometimes, this can be done through court orders requiring that things are done or not done. This ensures that clients receive the services to which they are entitled. Sometimes, the problems only come to light when it is too late, rights have been overridden or proper standards of care have not been met. Here, the law can only offer compensation for the victims of accidents.

It would be wrong for health professionals to assume that these functions mean that the law is a threat to their work.

In most areas it reinforces professional standards rather than undermines them. While the increase in litigation clearly brings genuine worries, the problems relate more to the financial consequences for health services than to restrictions on practitioners that prevent them exercising their clinical judgment in the best interests of their patients/clients. There are widely expressed worries about the phenomenon of defensive medicine. However, if this term describes health professionals doing things that they believe are against their clients' interests merely because the law requires it, then it is a myth. Such practices will not give health professionals better protection in law, because the law almost invariably requires them to achieve satisfactory standards as judged by their own peers and not by judges (Jones and Morris, 1989).

The corollary of the fact that the law reinforces basic professional standards is that staying within the law is not in itself a guarantee of ethical practice. The law marks out boundaries more than it determines what should happen. It tends to leave the professions to establish their own canons of ethics. Thus, awareness of the legal aspects of prenatal diagnosis will help professionals to avoid poor practice, but it cannot absolve them from grappling directly with the ethical issues. This chapter outlines the English legal framework within which prenatal diagnosis is carried out. It also considers briefly variations in other legal systems.

THE IMPACT OF THE LAW ON PRENATAL DIAGNOSIS

There are few legal rules designed specifically to solve the difficulties encountered in offering prenatal diagnosis. Instead, the implications of general principles need to be worked out. The law is therefore examined in relation to four stages in the process. The first is the making of decisions on whether to offer such testing. These will be taken at a macro level, when purchasers decide how far National Health Service funding will be made available for prenatal diagnosis. There will also be choices to be made about individual patients, choosing which tests (from among those that are possible) should be made available to them. The second stage in the process concerns the need for proper counselling if it is decided to offer testing. The third point at which legal standards are relevant concerns the testing itself.

Fourthly, it is necessary to consider the law governing the use of the results of prenatal diagnosis. This includes rules on the control of the information and also on the termination of pregnancy.

The provision of prenatal diagnosis

Under the National Health Service Act 1977 the Secretary of State for Health is obliged to provide a comprehensive health service. However, this does not mean that the National Health Service, or individual health professionals working within it, must provide everything possible. Nor does it mean that they must always give patients/clients what they want. Attempts to use the courts to force professionals to offer care when it does not have priority within existing resource constraints have consistently failed. Providing the decision is taken properly, with due care and without discrimination on the basis of the sex or race of the patient/client, it should be safe from legal challenge. Although these principles have not been tested in relation to services for prenatal diagnosis, they have been established in other contexts.

In 1980 a group of patients tried to use the courts to force a health authority and the Secretary of State to enhance orthopaedic services. It had been accepted that improvement was necessary and the Secretary of State had agreed to the building of a new hospital. However, the plans were then shelved due to lack of funding. The Court of Appeal rejected the patients' claim that the duty to provide a comprehensive health service had been breached. The judges stated that resource allocation was a political issue that was properly addressed through Parliament, not the courts (*R* v. *Secretary of State for Social Services*, ex p. *Hincks*, 1980). Thus, it appears that a purchaser who claimed that there was insufficient money to provide services for prenatal diagnosis would be safe from challenge through the courts.

Where the service is available, patients/clients may feel aggrieved if it is not offered to them. Such matters have also come to court. In 1987 a baby was being cared for in a Birmingham hospital while awaiting an operation to repair a hole in his heart. There were insufficient nursing staff to offer the operation to all the babies who would benefit from it. The parents of the baby sought an order from the court instructing the hospital to treat him. The Court of Appeal rejected their application. They

said that they could not get involved in the managerial questions
of resource allocation, nor could they rearrange waiting lists.
They would interfere only if a health authority acted wholly
unreasonably (*R* v. *Central Birmingham Health Authority*, ex p.
Walker, 1987).

There is little guidance as to what would be counted as an
unreasonable decision. The courts have indicated that it would
be improper to select patients on the basis of race (*R* v. *Ethical
Committee of St Mary's Hospital (Manchester)*, ex p. *Harriott*, 1988).
Presumably discrimination on the basis of sex would similarly
be unacceptable because, like racial discrimination, sex discrimination is prohibited by statute. It will usually be improper to
decide whether to offer prenatal diagnosis to people on the basis
of religious affiliation. Sometimes this is clear, as in the case of
Judaism, because the relevant religious group is also a racial one.
Nevertheless, even if it is not it would be unwise to rely on
religion as a determining factor.

This sort of factor may, of course, be important where a particular group wishes to use prenatal diagnosis as a way of pursuing
objectives (such as sex selection) that are unacceptable to health
professionals. It would be dangerous to refuse diagnostic testing
to patients/clients merely on the basis of their sex, religion or
race. This does not mean that there may not be acceptable reasons
for refusing to co-operate with such plans. In particular it may
be that in many cases there is no scope within the law for using
the information that would be generated. If sex alone could not
justify an abortion, then it would be proper to refuse testing on
the basis that it could not produce any usable information and
would thus be a waste of resources. The relevant aspects of
abortion law are discussed below.

These examples illustrate how reluctant the courts have proved
to be to interfere with managerial decisions on resource allocation
within the National Health Service. They have gone further still
in their deference to clinical judgment. While they have reserved
the right to override unreasonable decisions about the use of
resources, they have stated (in the context of the care of handicapped newborns) that doctors are entitled to 'refuse to adopt
treatment... on the basis that it is medically contraindicated or
for some other reason is a treatment which they could not con-
scientiously administer.' (Re J, 1990, p. 30). Even more explicitly,
it has also been held that it would be an abuse of the powers of

the courts to force a doctor to treat a patient against his/her clinical judgment (Re J, 1992). This principle would also be applied to cases outside the National Health Service.

The law previously described means that it would be very difficult indeed to obtain an order from a British court requiring that a patient be offered prenatal diagnosis. In practice, most challenges will be made after the event, alleging that the professional acted negligently, that is without reasonable care. That legal doctrine requires proof that the course of action taken would not be accepted as proper by a responsible body of professional people skilled in the area in question (*Bolam* v. *Friern Hospital Management Committee*, 1957). This effectively means that where the health professions believe that testing is inappropriate, then the law will allow them to withhold it from patients even when the patients are keen to have it. Where there are differing opinions within the professions, providing that the refusal to offer testing is acceptable to at least one school of thought it will not be negligent (*Maynard* v. *West Midlands Regional Health Authority*, 1983).

It should be noted that, where patient/clients are offered specialist services, they are entitled to expect that these will be properly carried out and that the standard of care is tailored to responsible professional practice in those specialties. Thus if prenatal diagnosis is offered it is no excuse for a mistake that some units could not offer such a service at all. Further, on this principle, hospitals as well as individual professionals may be liable if the services they deliver fail to meet the promised standard (*Wilsher* v. *Essex Area Health Authority*, 1988).

The net effect of these decisions of the English courts is that patients cannot demand prenatal diagnosis when health professionals genuinely and reasonably believe that it should be withheld. From one perspective this enables health professionals to protect patients from a self-destructive desire for knowledge at all costs. From another, it is paternalistic and permits health professionals to impose their views of the ethics of prenatal diagnosis on their patients/clients. In the private sector, the persuasive power of money may minimize the likelihood of this occurring. In the state-funded National Health Service it is an example of the general lack of patient power (Montgomery, 1994).

Counselling on testing

If it is decided to offer diagnostic testing, it will be necessary to obtain the consent of the person from whom the material to be tested will be obtained (Kennedy, 1992). Such a consent needs to be real, but in English law (in contrast to the position in many countries) it does not have to be fully informed. English law draws a distinction between the fact of consent to the procedure and the obligation to counsel patients. The former requires the patient to be informed in broad terms of what is to happen to them, to be capable of deciding to agree to it and to be free from coercion in doing so. A health professional may negate an otherwise valid consent by withholding information for improper reasons, but the failure to inform a patient/client of all the risks and alternatives will not usually render the test unlawful.

The extent of the duty to counsel patients/clients is determined by the test for negligence. This means that providing professional practice is followed there will be no scope for legal action. The courts have suggested that patients should normally be fully informed, especially if they ask questions, but have declined to set more precise legal standards for the health professions. Some guidance has been offered in the course of judicial discussion. Health professionals should be particularly diligent in informing patients of any special risks involved, that is risks which would (if they materialized) be particularly significant for them. The judges have also accepted that it is permissible to withhold information if it would harm the health of patients to reveal it. This guidance is not, however, legally binding. When the crunch comes, the courts have always returned to the professional standards test (Montgomery, 1988).

In practice, therefore, once again English law basically leaves the health professions to police themselves. It would almost certainly be negligent to fail to counsel a patient fully about the implications of prenatal diagnosis. However, this would be because professional opinion would regard a failure to counsel them as irresponsible, not because a judge has reached that conclusion.

Carrying out the test

Where prenatal diagnosis involves carrying out tests on the mother during pregnancy, then her consent will be sufficient to authorize it. However, where it involves preimplantation testing on gametes or embryos, it may need to be done under a licence from the Human Fertilisation and Embryology Authority. The Human Fertilisation and Embryology Act 1990 prohibits the storage of human gametes and the creation and storage of human embryos unless such a licence has been granted. Only if *in vitro* preimplantation testing is carried out on gametes without storing them will the need for a licence be avoided.

If the diagnostic test goes ahead, and something goes wrong, once again the legal action would be for negligence (Jones, 1992). This would be so whether the mishap was an inaccurate result, an injury to the child *in utero* or the loss of the baby. If there has been a genuine accident, without negligence, the action will fail. Proving that a medical accident during prenatal testing was the result of negligence would involve two stages. First, patients/clients would need to show that there had been an unacceptably poor standard of practice. Second, the person suing would have to prove that they had suffered 'damage' as a result of the mistake.

The first stage of the process involves the standard of care outlined above. The patient/client would have to prove that the person carrying out the tests had failed to meet the standards expected of them by their own peers. This does not mean that there must be uniform practice, but it means that the way in which the test was carried out must be regarded by experts from the profession as within the range of approaches that are regarded as legitimate. A mistake will constitute negligence if it is an error that would not have been made if responsible practice had been followed.

The courts have elaborated this test in a number of ways. It has already been pointed out that the courts will not prefer one accepted professional approach to another. The test for negligence is not designed to stifle innovation. Nor is it concerned with enforcing the best possible practice. Provided a minimum level of competence is attained, then the professional carrying out the tests has not been negligent.

The courts have also held that the victims of accidents should not lose out because the person caring for them is inexperienced. The hospital has an obligation to provide professional services and if they fail to do so they will be liable to compensate anybody who suffers injury as a result. Inexperienced hospital staff are expected to be competent to provide the services on offer but, if they are unsure of their skill, they may escape liability for accidents by recognizing their limitations and calling in more senior staff to confirm their diagnoses or carry out tricky procedures (*Wilsher* v. *Essex Area Health Authority,* 1988). Thus an individual practitioner may be protected from a negligence action, but the patient will still be compensated.

The second stage of a legal action, showing that damage was caused by the mistake, raises two issues. First, is the damage suffered something that the courts recognize as amenable to compensation through the law? Injury to the baby will qualify and the courts have accepted that the birth of an unwanted baby may also be damage for these purposes. Physical injury to the mother would also suffice, and pain and suffering that goes with it would also be compensated. However, distress alone, short of clinically diagnosed mental illness, is not compensated by English law. This would mean that, where an abnormality is falsely diagnosed, the woman (or couple) decide to continue with the pregnancy and a healthy infant is born, there would probably be little chance of a successful negligence action.

In practice, it will often be the case that the causal link between the injury suffered and the negligence will be unclear. It is for the person suing to prove the causal link and uncertainty will protect the professional. In essence the professional's defence would be that his/her mistake made no difference; any damage that the patient/client suffered would have occurred even without the mistake. The detailed application of this principle will vary according the type of case.

Where there is a failure to diagnose an abnormality, the court would need to consider whether anything could, or would, have been done to avoid the birth if the professionals had acted properly. If no legal abortion would have been available, even if a handicap had been detected, the chain of causation between mistake and injury would be broken. No action to prevent the birth could have been taken without breaking the law. Thus the birth of the disabled child would not have been a result of the mistake, but of the legal rules (*Rance* v. *Mid-Downs Health*

Authority, 1991). This makes the grounds for the termination of pregnancy (discussed below) significant in some negligence actions. Similarly, if the parents would not have chosen to terminate had they known the correct position, then the mistake would have made no difference.

Complications arise when the child is suing for errors in prenatal diagnosis. This cannot happen unless the child is born alive and there has been a breach of duty towards the mother (Congenital Disabilities (Liability) Act 1976). Even when this is the case, however, the courts have refused to accept claims for damages based on the claim that the person suing would rather not have been born at all (*McKay* v. *Essex Area Health Authority,* 1982). These are sometimes known as 'wrongful life' claims. Thus, a negligent failure to diagnose an abnormality or to counsel about the possibility of termination will not give rise to a legal action by the child. Where, however, a mistake in the diagnostic procedure actually causes an injury to the child, it may sue once it has been born.

Acting on the result

The first decision that has to be made once the results of prenatal diagnosis come through concerns informing the parents of the results. A distinction needs to be drawn between the obligations of health professionals to inform their patients/clients in response to specific questions and the rights of patients to seek information out. Failing to volunteer information would be legal unless the standard of care in negligence, as outlined above, was breached. It is therefore essentially a matter for the professions. However, it must be questionable whether professional practice would support testing when it was not intended to reveal the results. To fail to pass on the results of the test would thus probably be unlawful in many circumstances. The real problems arise when professionals wish to reveal some of the information obtained from prenatal testing, but not all of it. This raises the second issue.

Patients now have rights of access to their records. Where the records are held on computer this would be under the Data Protection Act 1984. Where the records are manual, the right of access is created by the Access to Health Records Act 1990 (in respect of records made after 1 November 1991). Neither of these

Acts creates absolute rights to see records in all circumstances. Access can be refused where it would be detrimental to the physical or mental health of the patient to allow it. Under the 1990 Act, but not the Data Protection Act 1984, access can also be denied on the basis that it would cause harm to the health of another person (other than the patient). However, as a fetus cannot generally constitute a legal person until it is born, it would not be possible to justify withholding the results of a test because they would be used to terminate a pregnancy. In order to avoid problems, health professionals might limit the amount of information recorded after tests to the minimum necessary for their clinical purposes.

This might become an issue where the test had been carried out to screen for an abnormality that the professional would have regarded as a legitimate ground for an abortion and that abnormality was excluded. Where the test also revealed other information that the patient/client (but not the professionals) regards as a ground for termination, there would be a dilemma. An obvious example would be the sex of the fetus. No professional could be forced to test for fetal sex against their wishes (see above). However, once the information is incorporated into the notes, patients will be entitled to see it on request unless the health professional responsible for their care can show that the patient's health would be at risk from having access to the facts.

A final legal issue in relation to the dissemination of the results of prenatal diagnosis concerns the position of the father of the fetus. Where testing has been carried out on a pregnant woman, technically the results are confidential to her. They should not, therefore, be passed on to her partner without her agreement. It would be safest to establish her views before carrying out the diagnostic tests. There would be no difficulty where tests are carried out on gametes or embryos *in vitro*, because both parents would be involved as patients (because the law requires both their consents).

The next decision to which the law is relevant concerns the possibility of abortion. There is no right to an abortion in English law. Rights imply entitlement, which is not secured by English law. The law establishes when abortions may be legal, and within those limits it makes two doctors the gatekeepers to the procedure (Abortion Act 1967, as amended by the Human Fertilisation and Embryology Act 1990). This means that a woman is never entitled to a termination of pregnancy, even when it would be lawful to carry one out. Professionals who oppose abortions on principle have an express legal right to opt out under the 'conscience clause' (Abortion Act 1967, s. 4). However, if a doctor believes that a particular woman's case is insufficiently meritorious she or he may simply decline to offer termination on the basis that the legal grounds have not been established. This point can be seen more clearly from an examination of the grounds set out in the Act.

Two of the four grounds on which terminations of pregnancy are legal may be in issue. They apply to selective reductions of multiple pregnancies as well as the termination of single pregnancies. The first is the so-called 'social ground' which is available up to 24 weeks. This covers cases where two doctors believe in good faith that the continuance of the pregnancy would involve risk, greater than if the pregnancy were terminated, of injury to the physical or mental health of the pregnant woman or any existing children of her family. The second is available until birth itself and covers cases where two doctors believe in good faith that there is a substantial risk that if the child were born it would suffer from such physical or mental abnormalities as to be seriously handicapped.

The precise meaning of each of these two grounds is unclear. It is sometimes argued that statistical evidence shows that it is always safer to terminate a pregnancy in the early stages than to carry the baby to term and deliver it. If this is the case, then there will always be a justification for abortions before the 24th week. No court has ever been asked to consider whether this approach would be legal. It is, however, clear that doctors have filled in the forms citing 'pregnancy' without more as the justification for abortions without being prosecuted. This 'statistical argument' could be used covertly to permit the abortion of fetuses of the undesired sex. It has also been argued that sex selection through termination of pregnancy may be openly practised on the basis that the woman would suffer ill-health due to the social stigma of having a baby of the 'wrong' sex (Morgan, 1988). Again, no court has had the opportunity to pronounce on the legality of such a practice.

The 'social grounds' for termination are available only before the end of the 24th week of pregnancy. Unfortunately, there is some doubt as to the way in which pregnancies are to be dated. Some commentators have suggested that the 24 weeks begin to run from the point of conception (Grubb, 1991; Murphy 1991). However, the best view is probably that the words refer to the usual clinical practice of dating from the first day of the woman's last menstrual period, correcting if necessary after an ultrasonic scan. This assumption is made by the Abortion Regulations 1991 (although the regulations cannot alter the meaning of the statute).

There is no time limit on terminations on the basis of fetal handicap. That ground is therefore available right up until the time of birth. However, it is unclear what degree of handicap would satisfy the test (Morgan, 1990). One case suggests that in essence the question is whether the child's life would be worth living (*McKay* v. *Essex Area Health Authority* 1982). Some help is given by the cases concerning the selective non-treatment of neonates. The courts have recognized that it is sometimes legitimate to withhold treatment, even though it is known that the result of doing so is likely to be the child's death. They have refused to authorize such a plan of care in relation to Down syndrome (Re B, 1981), but have accepted it where there was no prospect of prolonging the baby's life for any significant time (Re C, 1989). The Court of Appeal has also endorsed the decision of a paediatric team to decline to ventilate a child born very prematurely, severely brain-damaged and expected to be quadriplegic, blind, deaf and dumb (Re J, 1990). However, the courts have rejected suggestions that they should set out quasi-statutory guidelines on the degree of disability that would justify non-treatment. These decisions cannot really be taken to establish rules that the particular handicaps in issue would always be treated in the same way.

One of the implications of this uncertainty is that there is considerable scope for doctors to interpret the law so that it is line with their own moral views on what grounds provide an ethical justification for the termination of pregnancy. The legality of a termination does not actually depend on the precise meaning of (for example) 'seriously handicapped.' What matters is whether the doctors believed in good faith that this might be the case. Thus it is medical opinion which ultimately determines whether an abortion can be carried out and, unless it can be shown that the doctors acted in bad faith, it would be very difficult to impugn their decision.

CONCLUSION

This chapter has surveyed the main legal issues raised by pre-natal diagnosis. It has aimed to state the relevant principles of English law clearly, without becoming embroiled in the ethical problems discussed in the previous chapter. It has shown that in most areas the legal standards are determined by the health professions rather than the courts. The best way to avoid brushes with the law is therefore to pursue good professional practice. However, it is unlikely that the consciences of those practising prenatal diagnosis will be satisfied by merely avoiding legal difficulties. Staying within the boundaries of legally acceptable practice is no guarantee of good ethics. It may be the beginning of good ethical practice, but it is not enough.

The focus on English law has been deliberate because the degree of variation between legal systems is such that a compre-hensive survey would have to be of enormous length (see Giesen, 1988, for such a survey). The same four categories of legal prob-lem will arise in all systems. Access to services will be deter-mined largely by the way in which services are organized in the country in question. Where the provision is private, then it will rarely be possible to force a professional to offer tests, although malpractice laws may come close to doing so. In many countries of the world the legal standards required of health professionals in relation to both counselling and malpractice are more intrusive on clinical judgment. There is, therefore, no guarantee that other legal systems are so supportive of professional ethics as the English system. In relation to the grounds for termination of pregnancy, English law is neither particularly restrictive nor especially liberal (Glendon, 1987). The fundamental point, how-ever, is that each legal system must be considered in its own right.

By focusing on one system, that applied in England and Wales, the issues have been highlighted and the position in those coun-tries explained. This should enable English and Welsh prac-titioners to avoid legal problems. It should also assist those from other countries to discover their own laws by identifying the questions that they should ask.

REFERENCES

Bolam *v* Friern Hospital Management Committee (1957) 1 *Butterworths Medico-Legal Reports* 1–13.

Giesen, D (1988) *International Medical Malpractice Law*, Martinus Nijhoff Publications, Dordrecht, Holland.

Glendon, M.A. (1987) *Abortion and Divorce in Western Law*, Harvard University Press, Cambridge, MA.

Grubb, A. (1991) The new law of abortion: clarification or ambiguity? *Criminal Law Review* 659–670.

Jones, M.A. (1992) Medical Negligence, in *Doctors, Patients and the Law*, (ed. C. Dyer), Blackwell Scientific Publications, Oxford.

Jones, M.A. and Morris, A.E. (1989) Defensive medicine: myths and facts. *Journal of the Medical Defence Union*, **5**, 40–43.

Kennedy, I. (1992) Consent to treatment: the capable person, in *Doctors, Patients and the Law*, (ed. C. Dyer), Blackwell Scientific Publications, Oxford.

Maynard *v* West Midlands Regional Health Authority (1983) 1 *Butterworths Medico-Legal Reports* 122–131.

McKay *v* Essex Area Health Authority (1982) *Law Reports, Queens Bench* 1166.

Montgomery, J. (1988) Power/Knowledge/Consent: medical decision-making. *Modern Law Review* **51**, 245–255.

Montgomery, J. (1994) Patients first: the role of rights, in *Patient Centred Health Care*, (ed. K.W.M. Fulford, S. Erser and A. Hope), Blackwell Scientific Publications, Oxford, forthcoming.

Morgan, D. (1988) Foetal sex identification, abortion and the law. *Family Law* **18**, 355–359.

Morgan, D. (1990) Abortion: the unexamined ground. *Criminal Law Review* 687–694.

Murphy, J. (1991) Cosmetics, eugenics and ambivalence: the revision of the Abortion Act 1967. *Journal of Social Welfare and Family Law* 375–393.

R *v.* Central Birmingham Health Authority, *ex p.* Walker; R *v.* Secretary of State for Social Services, *ex p.* Walker (1987) 3 *Butterworths Medico-Legal Reports* 32–36.

R *v.* Ethical Committee of St Mary's Hospital (Manchester), *ex p.* Harriott, (1988) 1 *Family Law Reports* 512.

R *v.* Secretary of State for Social Services, West Midlands Regional Health Authority and Birmingham Area Health Authority, *ex p.* Hincks (1980) 1 *Butterworths Medico-Legal Reports* 93–97.

Rance *v.* Mid-Downs Health Authority (1991) 1 *All England Law Reports* 801–824.

Re B (1981) 1 *Weekly Law Reports* 1421–1425.

Re C (1989) 2 *All England Law Reports* 782–790.

Re J (1990) 6 *Butterworths Medico-Legal Reports* 25–43.

Re J (1992) 9 *Butterworths Medico-Legal Reports* 10–21.

Wilsher *v.* Essex Area Health Authority (1988) 3 *Butterworths Medico-Legal Reports* 37–91.

3

Women's experiences of prenatal screening and diagnosis

Josephine M. Green

INTRODUCTION

Although most pregnant women worry about the possibility that there might be something wrong with their baby, few have any specific grounds for this. Statham, Green and Snowdon (1992) found 'the possibility of something being wrong with the baby' to be one of the highest scoring worries in a sample of over 1800 women in early pregnancy, with only 11% being not at all worried. However, when asked 'Have you any reason to think that your baby might be more likely than any other to have some sort of a problem?' only 13% said 'yes', and these were primarily on grounds of age. Age is now widely recognized by women as a risk factor, which, as I shall argue below, may be a mixed blessing. Women take part in screening programmes in order to be reassured that their babies are healthy, rather than with any expectation that they are not and, as Farrant (1985) and Green, Snowdon and Statham (1993) have argued, it is important for service providers to appreciate the implications of this.

In this chapter I shall discuss what is known about women's experiences of prenatal screening and diagnosis, including findings from two major studies recently carried out in the United Kingdom. I shall conclude with some observations about the context of prenatal screening and, in particular, serum screening for Down syndrome. A full review of the literature on the psychological effects of fetal diagnosis on pregnant women can be found in Green (1990). This is particularly recommended for those who would like to understand more about the importance of methodological issues in this area.

DIAGNOSIS VERSUS SCREENING

In discussing diagnostic tests and screening tests different issues arise, so it is best to clarify the distinction before we start. Diagnostic tests are those that can give a (fairly) definitive answer to the question 'Does the baby have... (a particular disorder, e.g. spina bifida or Down syndrome)?'. If we had diagnostic tests for common disorders that were cheap and risk free, then we could apply them to everybody and we would not need screening tests. However, the reality is that the available diagnostic techniques (principally amniocentesis and chorionic villus sampling) are not cheap and they do carry a risk of miscarriage. It is therefore not considered appropriate for everybody to have them. Rather, we screen pregnant women to identify a subgroup which has a higher than average chance of having a baby with the disorder in question and for whom the costs and risks are therefore thought to be justified. The screening may be done on the basis of a woman's age, race or family history, or it may involve a screening test (e.g. measuring maternal serum alpha fetoprotein). Either way, screening *per se* can not tell us that the baby definitely does or does not have the disorder, only that there is a relatively high or low likelihood of that being the case. It is therefore in the nature of screening tests that they 'get it wrong', i.e. some people with a 'high risk' screening result (or 'screen positive') have babies that are fine ('false positive'), and some with a 'low risk' ('screen negative') do in fact have affected babies ('false negative'). Cut-offs are usually chosen to minimize the number of false negatives, but that often means a high proportion of false positives.

WOMEN'S EXPERIENCE OF DIAGNOSTIC TESTS

Women who have diagnostic tests fall into four groups: women who have had a previous handicapped child; women with a family history of a genetic disorder; women of 'advanced maternal age' (usually 35 plus); and women who have had positive screening tests. The two tests that we will consider in this chapter are amniocentesis, which is generally performed mid trimester at about 16 weeks, and chorionic villus sampling, which is performed at 10–12 weeks. Because it is done so early, chorionic villus sampling is only of use for risks which are known at the start of pregnancy, such as age and family history. Women whose risk is determined as a result of screening tests carried out during the pregnancy do not have this option.

Despite considerable methodological variation (Green, 1990), some consistent findings about women's experiences of amniocentesis emerge from the literature. These concern worries about potential miscarriage and the stressful nature of the 3–4 week waiting period for results, followed, usually, by a drop in anxiety once normal results are given. The first controlled study comparing women having amniocentesis with women who were not (Fava *et al.*, 1982, 1983) found no differences between the groups by mid-pregnancy and therefore concluded that amniocentesis does not allay anxiety. Three subsequent studies (Phipps and Zinn, 1986; Marteau, 1991; Statham, Green and Snowdon, 1992) have also failed to find significantly lower anxiety scores for women who have had negative amniocentesis results compared to untested controls. The latter two studies have concluded that differences between groups are likely to relate to pre-existing characteristics, which is a recurring theme in this area (Green, 1990).

Comparison of women aged less than 35 who were allocated to having amniocentesis without any particular indication for the procedure with those having amniocentesis on the grounds of their age (Tabor and Jonsson, 1987) showed a decline in anxiety for the younger women immediately after the procedure while for older women it did not drop until normal results had been given. Another Scandinavian study (Sjogren and Uddenberg, 1990) found that younger women who were having prenatal diagnosis because of self-reported anxiety were actually not particularly anxious once their request for the test had been granted. As one said: 'Now, when I am allowed to have the test, I don't worry about what will follow.' These findings underline the other main message that emerges from the literature which is that the main determinant of women's reactions to the process of prenatal diagnosis is the reason for having it.

As early as 1975, Robinson, Tennes and Robinson, reporting

on women having amniocentesis on the grounds of their age, stated that they 'saw the test as an appropriate part of intelligent prenatal care and expected a benign outcome'. Evers-Kiebooms, Swerts and van den Berghe (1988) compared women having amniocentesis for maternal age with those who had had a previous child with Down syndrome or a neural tube defect. Mothers of Down syndrome children were most anxious while waiting for the results, while those who had previous experience of a neural tube defect were the ones least likely to be reassured by a negative result. Other studies have also generally shown that women who previously have had affected children are more anxious and less likely to be reassured, while women being tested simply on grounds of age are the least anxious (e.g. Chervin *et al.*, 1977; Beeson and Golbus, 1979). However, the literature also shows very clearly another group for whom amniocentesis is particularly stressful: those having amniocentesis because of raised alpha fetoprotein levels (see below). Farrant (1980) showed that, in contrast to the situation described for older women, amniocentesis was not viewed as a routine component of antenatal care, rather it was seen as part of a relentless process challenging what was previously believed to be a normal pregnancy.

The assumption has always been that chorionic villus sampling would be less stressful for women than amniocentesis for three reasons.

- They do not have to wait so long to have the test done (10 weeks after their last period instead of 16).
- They do not have to wait so long for results (one week versus three or four).
- Termination of pregnancy, if indicated, can be carried out in the first trimester and thus by dilatation and curettage rather than by inducing labour at 20 weeks or more.

The first two assumptions are, on the whole, supported by the literature. McCormack *et al.* (1990), for example, in a retrospective study of 152 women who had had chorionic villus sampling, found high acceptability and willingness to accept higher miscarriage rates as a trade-off for the benefits of earlier and quicker results. This was especially true for women at known risk of passing on a genetic disorder. Data are lacking with respect to the third assumption, that earlier terminations are less distressing. The only relevant studies (Black, 1989; Robinson *et al.*, 1991) are too small and methodologically confused to allow conclusions to be drawn (see also Chapter 11).

The first study comparing experiences of chorionic villus sampling and amniocentesis involved 61 women enrolled in the Canadian randomized control trial (Spencer and Cox, 1987, 1988). Robinson *et al.* (1988) published a separate study, based on another 54 women from the same trial. Both studies indicated that chorionic villus sampling evoked less anxiety over a shorter period of time than amniocentesis. Spencer and Cox reported that women having amniocentesis were suppressing their attachment to their fetus until after they had had a negative result. Robinson *et al.* did not measure attachment until 22 weeks, at which point there was no difference between the groups. However, they subsequently investigated a different set of women, who were not part of the trial (Caccia *et al.*, 1991), and did find that attachment scores rose after a reassuring test result, whether this was at 15 weeks (for the chorionic villus sampling group) or at 21 weeks (for the amniocentesis group). This finding may be taken as support for Barbara Katz Rothman's idea of the 'tentative pregnancy' (Rothman, 1986). Kolker (1989) suggests that these 'positive' feelings after negative test results are a function of the anxiety created by the test itself: had the test not raised anxieties, there would be no need for reassurance. This interpretation is consistent with the findings from the amniocentesis studies quoted above that found no net benefit to tested women compared to those who were not tested.

In evaluating the data in this area, it is important to know whether women are undergoing a procedure that they have chosen or whether they have been randomized. Verjaal, Leschot and Treffers (1982) showed that women who actively sought amniocentesis start from a position of greater commitment to the procedure and are likely to be loyal to their choice. The irony of randomized trials is that they can create differences between groups: those that get what they want versus those that do not. In Britain, for example, the trial comparing amniocentesis and chorionic villus sampling got off to a very slow start because most women did not want to be randomized (MacKenzie, Boyd and Ferguson, 1986). Having been counselled as to the two methods, they had formed a preference and did not want their fate decided by the toss of a coin. To tolerate the delays and anxieties of amniocentesis when everyone else is in the same boat is one thing; to tolerate them in the knowledge that you could have had your results 10 weeks sooner, had you been otherwise randomized, is quite different. That women did have more negative feelings about amniocentesis in this context is clear from the Spencer and Cox study where 100% of the 31 women planning further pregnancies said that they would want chorionic villus sampling next time. In contrast, another study (Tunis *et al.*, 1990), which compared 30 women who had chosen to have amniocentesis with 151 who had chosen chorionic villus sampling, found virtually no differences between the groups on a range of psychological indices, in direct contrast to the findings on women enrolled in the trials.

There is one other important point to be made about chorionic villus sampling versus amniocentesis, which is raised by Robinson *et al.* (1991) concerning miscarriage after chorionic villus sampling. Compared with amniocentesis, a relatively large number of women will miscarry after chorionic villus sampling, partly because it does actually cause more miscarriages than amniocentesis and partly because there is a higher rate of spontaneous loss at this earlier stage of pregnancy. However, no one can know whether their particular miscarriage was a consequence of the procedure or was one that would have happened anyway. Robinson *et al.* found that women who miscarried after chorionic villus sampling experienced a great deal of guilt and blamed their loss on their selfish desire for an earlier test result. In fact, they had even less reason for feeling this way than might be supposed because they were part of the randomized trial and had not actually chosen to have chorionic villus sampling. This is an important point which should be taken into account when counselling women for prenatal diagnosis. Related to it is the higher rate of terminations of pregnancy for fetal chromosomal anomaly following chorionic villus sampling compared with amniocentesis (MRC Working Party on the Evaluation of Chorionic Villus Sampling, 1991). The working party was, unfortunately, not able to say how many of these were false positives because post-termination karyotyping was not always carried out. Neither, of course, were they able to say how many true positives would have aborted spontaneously before the 16th week. Either way, the higher termination rate is another risk of the procedure that women should be aware of.

WOMEN'S EXPERIENCE OF SERUM SCREENING

Maternal serum alpha fetoprotein screening for neural tube defects has been in common use in the United Kingdom since the late 1970s. More recently it has also been used to screen for Down syndrome. The test is usually carried out at 16 weeks. As a screening test (see above), it necessarily has false positives and false negatives. The test's accuracy depends critically on gestational age being correctly known since the level of alpha fetoprotein increases by about 19% per week in the second trimester (Wald and Cuckle, 1984).

There are two questions that might reasonably be addressed by research in this area: what are the psychological effects on women who have a false positive screening result and what are the effects on women whose result is normal? The second question has received somewhat less attention than the first. A Swedish study (Berne-Fromell, Kjessler and Josefson, 1983; Berne-Fromell and Kjessler, 1984), and an American study (Burton, Dillard and Clark, 1985a) have both addressed the question, but in each case there are methodological difficulties which make the results difficult to interpret (Green, 1990). Both cautiously concluded that any differences between screened and unscreened women were minor, favoured the screened women and did not suggest long-term harm resulting from participation in the screening programme. Two recent British studies have also considered this issue. The first (Marteau *et al.*, 1992a) was carried out in one London hospital where the test is routine. Unscreened women were therefore likely to be atypical and to differ from those having the test and indeed, women who declined testing were found to differ from those who were simply omitted. The Cambridge Prenatal Screening Study (Green, Statham and Snowdon, 1994) compared women both within and between groups of hospitals that did or did not offer routine alpha fetoprotein screening. Here it was found that untested women in hospitals where the test was routine were significantly less worried about something being wrong with the baby, and this difference existed before the test was offered. Thus the conclusion would seem to be that the test was not **causing** higher anxiety, but was being accepted by those who were more anxious initially. This was also the conclusion of Marteau *et al*. This interpretation is supported by the further finding from the Cambridge study that tested women were neither more nor less worried than women in hospitals where the test was not offered (Statham, Green and Snowdon, 1992). In other words, while the test was not generating worries, neither did it seem to be allaying them, although both studies do suggest the possibility of lower anxiety in tested women in late pregnancy. A further finding from the Cambridge study, which suggests that this test has now become a non-event for many women in the United Kingdom, was that there were no differences in the worries of women who had been 'told the result was normal' compared with those who 'haven't been told, but assume it's all right.'

The effects of false positive alpha fetoprotein results were first reported by Farrant (1980) and Fearn *et al.* (1982), who both found exceedingly high levels of anxiety. Fearn *et al.* found that the anxiety persisted even when the women were told that there was not a problem after all. The most severe levels of anxiety were found in women who, having gone on to have amniocentesis, were not told the results. They were just told to assume that all was well if they did not hear to the contrary. It is to be hoped that this practice no longer occurs.

The finding that abnormal alpha fetoprotein results create anxiety has been confirmed in all subsequent studies (Berne-Fromell, Uddenberg and Kjessler, 1983; Burton, Dillard and Clark 1985b; Marteau *et al.*, 1992b; Green, Statham and Snowdon, 1994). The largest study (Burton, Dillard and Clark, 1985b) involved an initial sample of over 6000 women, 205 of whom were found to have elevated alpha fetoprotein and 179 of whom agreed to participate. Control subjects were selected from women with normal alpha fetoprotein tested on the same day and matched, if possible, for race, age and parity. Interestingly, control subjects were found to be of higher social class. All participants completed anxiety and attitude to pregnancy scales prior to testing and on eleven subsequent occasions. Anxiety was very high in women with abnormal alpha fetoprotein and did not drop until after normal results had been given. Thereafter scores were very similar for all subjects and controls. There was no evidence of residual anxiety for the women with initially raised alpha fetoprotein.

Most published studies have been concerned with alpha fetoprotein screening for neural tube defects, but there have been a small number of reports of women's experiences of serum screening for Down syndrome. The first preliminary report came from Marteau *et al.* (1988), indicating that younger women (under 38) experience very high levels of anxiety even after receiving subsequent normal results, while older women, who are nowadays encouraged to think of themselves as being at higher risk for Down syndrome, show similar levels of anxiety whether or not their alpha fetoprotein levels are low. This is a somewhat surprising finding suggesting that the older women may not have understood the implications of the low alpha fetoprotein results. Other studies have confirmed that low alpha fetoprotein results cause considerable distress (Evans *et al.*, 1988; Abuelo *et al.*, 1991; Keenan *et al.*, 1991; Roelofsen, Kamerbeek and Tymstra, 1993). The State Anxiety scores (Spielberger, Gorsuch and Lushene, 1970) reported by Keenan *et al.* for women with **low** alpha fetoprotein levels are much higher than the comparable scores reported by Burton, Dillard and Clark (1985b) for women with **high** alpha fetoprotein levels. A number of authors (e.g. Abuelo *et al.*, 1991) have specifically drawn attention to the higher anxiety of women selected as 'high risk' for Down syndrome on the basis of a serum screening test in contrast to those with the identical numerical risk based on age alone. The extent of this in Abuelo's study was that 'several women with low alpha fetoproteins refused to participate in our study because they stated that they were 'too nervous'' (p. 384).

The use of alpha fetoprotein screening to identify younger women at risk of Down syndrome is now being superseded by serum screening which uses additional biochemical markers to give better definition of the at risk population (Wald *et al.*, 1988). This is causing confusion and anxiety both to pregnant women (Statham and Green, 1993) and to staff, as has been clear at numerous recent meetings (e.g. Kings Fund, 13 July 1992). It was predicted that the triple test would detect 60% of Down syndrome fetuses with an amniocentesis rate of 5%. Screening based on age alone detects, at best, 35% of cases and involves 7–8% of the population (i.e. all women aged 35 or over) having amniocentesis. Thus triple testing should mean fewer women subjected to the stress of amniocentesis and more affected fetuses detected. However, as Donnai and Andrews (1988) predicted, the idea that being over 35 puts a woman at risk for Down syndrome is now so well established that these older women are unwilling to lose their 'right' to diagnostic testing. Roelofsen, Kamerbeek and

Tymstra (1993) found that 55% of 155 older mothers in the Netherlands would want serum screening for Down syndrome in a subsequent pregnancy, but 76% of them would still want amniocentesis, even if they were found to be 'low risk'.

WOMEN'S EXPERIENCE OF ULTRASOUND SCANNING

Ultrasound scanning is in a different category from other techniques for investigating fetal wellbeing. Firstly, it gives instant results – the process is happening there and then. Secondly, it does not fit easily into a classification of 'screening' versus 'diagnosis'. In the sense that it is used on everybody (in the United Kingdom), irrespective of risk status 'just to make sure that the baby is all right', it is being used as a screening technique. It may reveal findings that are of limited significance in their own right but are known to be associated with certain syndromes. In these cases the scan findings will be the cue for further diagnostic investigations. This is increasingly happening for chromosomal disorders (Nicolaides *et al.*, 1992). However, scans may also give definitive information about, for example, structural abnormalities, number of fetuses and fetal death, so in this sense they are diagnostic. The studies that will be discussed here are those concerned with routine scanning of low risk women. The experiences of high risk women and those who have abnormalities detected via ultrasound scans have been described elsewhere (Green, 1990; Green, Statham and Snowdon, 1992).

When ultrasound scans were first introduced into antenatal care they were (supposedly) only used when the obstetrician suspected that there might be a problem and women were not allowed to see the screen. I have my own memories of being forcibly held down to prevent me from seeing the screen, and in those early days being sent for a scan elicited sympathy. Endless waiting with a full bladder was considered a form of torture that only a true misogynist would have dreamt up for pregnant women. Everything changed once women were allowed to see the screen.

Studies of women's experiences of ultrasound from the early 1980s, e.g. Milne and Rich (1981) and the Kings College Hospital study (Reading and Cox, 1982; Campbell *et al.*, 1982; Reading *et al.*, 1982) showed that what women liked about scans was a moving image that was interpreted for them. Nowadays that is what women expect. For most British women, 'seeing' the baby on the scan is a high spot of the pregnancy, an event to be shared with the baby's father and siblings. We asked the women in the Cambridge Prenatal Screening Study if they felt that they could have said 'no' to the scan. Many clearly found this an extraordinary question: why should they wish to say no? Roberts (1986) found that the scan operator was the single most important determinant of women's satisfaction with the scan. However, to quote from Campbell *et al*. 'In busy clinics, insufficient attention may be given to providing feedback and in some cases reassurance'. We see the evidence of this, not from studies that are focused on ultrasound, but from those which have retrospectively sampled (and thus not altered) everyday practice. Jacoby (1988), for example, quotes one woman's experience of ultrasound: 'I was not spoken to. The scan was not explained and my questions were totally ignored. I felt I was just a nuisance, and was sure something was wrong with the child as the comments written were placed in a large firmly sealed envelope...'.

Similar comments were given by some mothers in Hyde's (1986) study. 'I've seen it on television, and I was led to believe it would be explained.' 'You build yourself up, then they don't say anything.' Hyde's study is of considerable interest because it was carried out in the United Kingdom during the very small time window when ultrasound scanning was becoming common but was not yet the norm. She found that unscanned women in hospitals where ultrasound was not used routinely were less likely to see scans as a source of reassurance. This would seem to be a classic example of the belief that 'what **is** must be best' as observed by Porter and Macintyre (1984).

When Hyde was carrying out her survey in 1982, many women were still very suspicious of this new technology. Nowadays, women's main complaint about ultrasound in pregnancy – as we found in the Cambridge Prenatal Screening Study – is that they do not get enough of it. However, an interesting report from another recent study suggests that the suspicion of ultrasound is not in fact so far below the surface. Thorpe *et al*. (1993) asked mothers of newborn children about their views of ultrasound scanning in a non-routine context: cerebral scanning of neonates. Many mothers had misgivings about this which they then had to accommodate within their framework of acceptance of antenatal scanning, for example: 'I know it's not harmful through me – it is just the thought of doing it on him.' 'She is only a baby, she's not old enough to have one whereas I am.'

One of the most telling comments from Thorpe's respondents was 'This [cerebral] scan looks for things that are wrong whereas the scan in pregnancy checks to see that the baby is OK.' This distinction between 'checking that everything is OK' and 'looking for abnormalities' is probably one of the keys to women's enthusiasm for scans: they do not view them as a threat that might give them bad news (like amniocentesis) but as a benign procedure that allows them to see their baby and confirm that it is healthy. Their assumption that the procedure is benign is, of course, encouraged by the fact that scans are routine and given to everyone. Thus, to quote another of Thorpe's subjects: 'If it was necessary I would have [consented] – if it was routine – no problem.'

CONCLUSIONS

Prenatal screening and diagnosis do not happen in a vacuum, and a woman's experiences are related to both the broad societal context (Green, Statham and Snowdon, 1992) and the more specific circumstances that have led her to be having this test at this time. Perhaps the most neglected of these circumstances has been the historical context. As we see from the literature, women react differently to tests that are new compared to those that are accepted as routine procedures (Richards and Green, 1993). This is likely to be a partial explanation of the current difficulties being experienced with serum screening for Down syndrome. In addition, the test is a development of an existing test (alpha fetoprotein screening for neural tube defects), so that people think that they know what it is. It is also replacing (at least in theory) another method of screening – age – which is not actually recognized by most people as being a screening test at all. So effective has been the message that older women are at risk for chromosomal abnormalities that the fact that two-thirds of Down syndrome babies are born to younger women has been buried.

Another source of confusion is that serum screening results are frequently reported as risk figures: 'one in so-and-so-many', which people find difficult to interpret. They want to know 'Is this the "one" or isn't it?'. Notwithstanding the history of alpha fetoprotein screening for neural tube defects in this country, the concept of a screening test which necessarily has false positives and false negatives is poorly understood. The positive predictive value of the triple test is 1 in 68, in other words 67 out of every 68 women who screen positive will not have an affected baby (this compares with figures for neural tube defect serum screening varying from 1 in 15 to 1 in 66, depending on incidence). Using age alone as the screening method for Down syndrome has considerably poorer positive predictive value. Even at age 40, when the risk is 1 in 110, that still means that 109 out of 110 40-year-olds have been selected for amniocentesis but do not have an affected baby. It may be that the poor predictive value of age is one of the factors which makes it a less threatening screening method: a woman selected for amniocentesis on the basis of her age is, on average, only half as likely to have a Down syndrome baby as one selected by serum screening. However, it is likely that the other factor that makes serum screening so much more alarming to women is the fact that it is based on specific information about this particular pregnancy, not just membership of an impersonal risk group.

While the passage of time will undoubtedly solve some of the problems currently being experienced with serum screening for Down syndrome, many will remain that need to be addressed by better education of both staff and pregnant women and by a greater appreciation of psychological factors.

REFERENCES

Abuelo, D.N., Hopmann, M.R., Barsel-Bowers, G. and Goldstein, A. (1991) Anxiety in women with low maternal serum alpha-fetoprotein screening results. *Prenatal Diagnosis*, **11**: 381–385.

Beeson, D. and Golbus, M.S. (1979) Anxiety engendered by amniocentesis. *Birth Defects Original Articles Series*, **15**, 191–197.

Berne-Frommel, K., Kjessler, B. and Josefson, G. (1983) Anxiety concerning fetal malformation in women who accept or refuse alpha-fetoprotein screening in pregnancy. *Journal of Psychosomatic Obstetrics and Gynaecology*, **2**, 94–97.

Berne-Fromell, K., Uddenberg, N. and Kjessler, B. (1983) Psychological reactions experienced by pregnant women with an elevated serum alpha-fetoprotein level. *Journal of Psychosomatic Obstetrics and Gynaecology*, **2**, 233–237.

Berne-Frommel, K. and Kjessler, B. (1984) Anxiety concerning fetal malformations in pregnant women exposed or not exposed to an antenatal serum alpha-fetoprotein screening program. *Gynecologic and Obstetric Investigation*, **17**, 36–39.

Black, R.B. (1989) A 1 and 6 month follow-up of prenatal diagnosis patients who lost pregnancies. *Prenatal Diagnosis*, **9**, 795–804.

Burton, B.K., Dillard, R.G. and Clark, E.N. (1985a) Maternal serum alpha-fetoprotein screening: the effect of participation on anxiety and attitude toward pregnancy in women with normal results. *American Journal of Obstetrics and Gynecology*, **152**, 540–543.

Burton, B.K., Dillard, R.G. and Clark, E.N. (1985b) The psychological impact of false positive elevations of maternal serum alpha-fetoprotein. *American Journal of Obstetrics and Gynecology*, **151**, 77–82.

Caccia, N., Johnson, J.M., Robinson, G.E. and Barna, T. (1991) Impact of prenatal testing on maternal-fetal bonding: chorionic villus sampling versus amniocentesis. *American Journal of Obstetrics and Gynecology* **165**:(4), 1122–1125.

Campbell, S., Reading, A.E., Cox, D.N. *et al.* (1982) Ultrasound scanning in pregnancy. *Journal of Psychosomatic Obstetrics and Gynecology*, **1**, 57–61.

Chervin, A., Farnsworth, P.B., Freedman, W.L. *et al.* (1977) Amniocentesis for prenatal diagnosis. *New York State Journal of Medicine*, **August**, 1406–1408.

Donnai, D. and Andrews, T. (1988) Screening for Down's syndrome. New methods allow detection of three fifths of affected pregnancies. *British Medical Journal*, **297**, 876.

Evans, M.I., Bottoms, S.F., Carlucci, T. *et al.* (1988) Determinants of altered anxiety after abnormal maternal serum alpha-fetoprotein screening. *American Journal of Obstetrics and Gynecology*, **159**, 1501–1504.

Evers-Kiebooms, G., Swerts, A. and van den Berghe, H. (1988) Psychological aspects of amniocentesis: anxiety feelings in three different risk groups. *Clinical Genetics*, **33**, 196–206.

Farrant, W. (1980) Stress after amniocentesis for high serum alpha-fetoprotein concentrations. *British Medical Journal*, **281**, 452.

Farrant, W. (1985) 'Who's for amniocentesis?' The politics of prenatal screening, in *The Sexual Politics of Reproduction*, (ed. H. Homans), Gower, London.

Fava, G.A., Kellner, R., Michelacci, L. *et al.* (1982) Psychological reactions to amniocentesis: a controlled study. *American Journal Obstetrics and Gynecology*, **143**, 509–513.

Fava, G.A., Trombini, G., Michelacci, L. *et al.* (1983) Hostility in women before and after amniocentesis. *Journal of Reproductive Medicine*, **28**, 29–34.

Fearn, J., Hibbard, B.M., Roberts, A. *et.al.* (1982) Screening for neural-tube defects and maternal anxiety. *British Journal of Obstetrics and Gynaecology*, **89**, 218–221.

Green, J.M. (1990) Calming or harming: a critical review of psychological effects of fetal diagnosis on pregnant women. *Galton Institute Occasional Papers*, Second series, No 2.

Green, J.M., Snowdon, C. and Statham, H. (1993) Pregnant women's

References   *51*

attitudes to abortion and prenatal screening. *Journal of Reproductive and Infant Psychology,* **11**, 31–39.

Green, J.M., Statham, H. and Snowdon, C. (1992) Screening for fetal abnormalities: attitudes and experiences, in *Obstetrics in the 1990s: Current Controversies,* (eds T. Chard and M.P.M. Richards), McKeith Press, London, pp. 65–89.

Green, J.M., Statham, H. and Snowdon, C. (1994) *Pregnancy: A Testing Time,* Report of the Cambridge Prenatal Screening Study, Centre for Family Research, University of Cambridge, Cambridge.

Hyde, B. (1986) An interview study of pregnant women's attitudes to ultrasound scanning. *Social Science and Medicine,* **22**, 587–592.

Jacoby, A. (1988) Mothers' views about information and advice in pregnancy and childbirth: findings from a national study. *Midwifery,* **4**, 103–110.

Keenan, K.L., Basso, D., Goldkrand, J. and Butler, W.J. (1991) Low level of maternal serum alpha-fetoprotein: its associated anxiety and the effects of genetic counselling. *American Journal of Obstetrics and Gynecology,* **164**, 54–56.

Kolker, A. (1989) Advances in prenatal diagnosis: social-psychological and policy issues. *International Journal of Technology Assessment in Health Care,* **5**, 601–617.

McCormack, M.J., Rylance, M.E., Newton, J. *et al.* (1990) Patients' attitudes following chorionic villus sampling. *Prenatal Diagnosis,* **10**, 253–255.

MacKenzie, I.Z., Boyd, P. and Ferguson, J. (1986) Chorion villus sampling and randomization. *Lancet,* **26 April**, 969–970.

Marteau, T.M. (1991) Psychological aspects of prenatal testing for fetal abnormalities. *Irish Journal of Psychology,* **12**, 121–132.

Marteau, T.M., Kidd, J., Cook, R. *et al.* (1988) Screening for Down's syndrome. *British Medical Journal,* **297**, 1469.

Marteau, T.M., Johnson, M., Kidd, J. *et al.* (1992a) Psychological models in predicting uptake of prenatal screening. *Psychology and Health,* **6**, 13–22.

Marteau, T.M., Cook, R., Kidd, J. *et al.* (1992b) The psychological effects of false positive results in prenatal screening for fetal abnormality: a prospective study. *Prenatal Diagnosis,* **12**, 205–214.

Milne, L.S. and Rich, U.J. (1981) Cognitive and affective aspects of the responses of pregnant women to sonography. *Maternal–Child Nursing Journal (Pittsburg),* **10**, 15–39.

MRC Working Party on the Evaluation of Chorion Villus Sampling (1991) MRC European trial of chorion villus sampling. *Lancet,* **337**, 1491–1499.

Nicolaides, K.H., Snijders, R.J.M., Gosden, C.M. *et al.* (1992) Ultrasonographically detectable markers of fetal chromosomal abnormalities. *Lancet,* **340**, 704–707.

Phipps, S. and Zinn, A.B. (1986) Psychological response to amniocentesis: I. Mood state and adaptation to pregnancy. *American Journal of Medical Genetics,* **25**, 131–142.

Porter, M. and Macintyre, S. (1984) What is, must be best: a research note on conservative or deferential responses to antenatal care provision. *Social Science and Medicine*, **19**(11), 1197–1200.

Reading, A.E., Campbell, S., Cox, D.N. and Sledmore, C.M. (1982) Health beliefs and health care behaviour in pregnancy. *Psychological Medicine*, **12**, 379–383.

Reading, A.E. and Cox, D.N. (1982) The effects of ultrasound examination on maternal anxiety levels. *Journal of Behavioral Medicine*, **5**, 237–247.

Richards, M.P.M. and Green, J.M. (1993) Attitudes toward prenatal screening for fetal abnormality and detection of carriers of genetic disease: a discussion paper. *Journal of Reproductive and Infant Psychology*, **11**, 49–56.

Roberts, J. (1986) The consumer's viewpoint on ultrasound in pregnancy. *Bulletin of the British Medical Ultrasound Society*, Feb/Mar, 18–19.

Robinson, G.E., Carr, M.L., Olmsted, M.P. and Wright, C. (1991) Psychological reactions to pregnancy loss after prenatal diagnostic testing: preliminary results. *Journal of Psychosomatic Obstetrics and Gynaecology*, **12**, 181–192.

Robinson, G.E., Garner, D.M., Olmstead, M.P. *et al.* (1988) Anxiety reduction after chorionic villus sampling and genetic amniocentesis. *American Journal of Obstetrics and Gynecology*, **159**, 953–956.

Robinson, J., Tennes, K. and Robinson, A. (1975) Amniocentesis: its impact on mothers and infants. A 1-year follow-up study. *Clinical Genetics*, **8**, 97–106.

Roelofsen, E.E.C., Kamerbeek, L.I. and Tymstra, T.J. (1993) Chances and choices. Psycho-social consequences of maternal serum screening. A report from the Netherlands. *Journal of Reproductive and Infant Psychology*, **11**, 41–47.

Rothman, B.K. (1986) *The Tentative Pregnancy: Prenatal Diagnosis and the Future of Motherhood*, Viking Penguin, New York.

Sjogren, B. and Uddenberg, N. (1990) Prenatal diagnosis for psychological reasons: comparison with other indications, advanced maternal age and known genetic risk. *Prenatal Diagnosis*, **10**, 111–120.

Spencer, J.W. and Cox, D.N. (1987) Emotional responses of pregnant women to chorionic villi sampling or amniocentesis. *American Journal of Obstetrics and Gynecology*, **157**, 1155–1160.

Spencer, J.W. and Cox, D.N. (1988) A comparison of chorionic villi sampling and amniocentesis: acceptability of procedure and maternal attachment to pregnancy. *Obstetrics and Gynecology*, **72**, 714–718.

Spielberger, C.D., Gorsuch, R.L. and Lushene, R.E. (1970) *The State–Trait Anxiety Inventory*. Consulting Psychologists Press, .

Statham, H. and Green, J. (1993) Serum screening for Down's syndrome: some women's experiences. *British Medical Journal*, **307**, 174–176.

Statham, H., Green, J. and Snowdon, C. (1992) Psychological and social aspects of screening for fetal abnormality during routine antenatal care, in *Proceedings of 'Research and the Midwife'*, November 1992.

Tabor, A., Jonsson, M.H. (1987) Psychological impact of amniocentesis in low risk women. *Prenatal Diagnosis*, **7**, 443–449.

Thorpe, K., Harker, L., Pike, A. and Marlow, N. (1993) Women's views of ultrasonography: a comparison of women's experiences of antenatal ultrasound screening with cerebral ultrasound of their newborn infant. *Social Science and Medicine*, **36**, 311–315.

Tunis, S.L., Golbus, M.S., Copeland, K.L. *et al.* (1990) Patterns of mood states in pregnant women undergoing chorionic villus sampling or amniocentesis. *American Journal of Medical Genetics*, **37**, 191–199.

Verjaal, M., Leschot, N.J. and Treffers, P.E. (1982) Women's experiences with second trimester prenatal diagnosis. *Prenatal Diagnosis*, **2**, 195–209.

Wald, N.J. and Cuckle, H.S. (1984) Open neural-tube defects, in *Antenatal and Neonatal Screening*, (ed. N.J. Wald), Oxford University Press, Oxford.

Wald, N.J., Cuckle, H.S., Densem, J.W. *et al.* (1988) Maternal serum screening for Down's syndrome in early pregnancy. *British Medical Journal*, **297**, 883–887.

4

Screening issues – the public health aspect

Jean Chapple

Public health specialists differ from nurses and doctors involved in clinical medicine in that their 'patients' are whole communities rather than the individuals who make up that community. This creates a potential tension between those making health policy decisions which affect society as a whole and those who have day to day contact with individuals and who need resources to deliver that clinical care. In general, what is good for the individual is also good for society, but this is not inevitably the case. Diagnosing and treating one person may mean that no resources are left to diagnose and treat another. These are the opportunity costs of a programme and mean that Dr Paul may be robbing Dr Peter of his/her chance to treat the patient sitting in front of them (Mooney, 1992). This chapter looks at some of the difficulties in running screening and diagnostic programmes while ensuring that the individuals who look to health services are treated as people and not as inanimate products on a eugenic production line.

Public health has been defined as the science and art of preventing disease, prolonging life and promoting health through the organized efforts of society (Acheson, 1988). Public health has five main roles to play in prenatal diagnosis and screening:

- assessing when and why malformations occur;
- assessing the need for screening;
- evaluating pilot screening projects;

- informing public policy decisions about screening;
- monitoring the results of population screening programmes.

ASSESSING WHEN AND WHY MALFORMATIONS OCCUR

The core science of public health is epidemiology, the study of the distribution and determinants of disease. This means looking at data from large populations to see what malformations occur, how often they occur and who is affected.

Congenital malformations are generally rare, about 2% of all fetuses having a major malformation. The average general practitioner who looks after about 3000 patients will have no more than 60 new babies in the practice each year and would expect to see fewer than one baby a year with a major genetic problem. If a new health hazard arises which doubles the rate of malformations, it is easy to see that the general practitioner would regard two babies with malformations in a year as entirely due to chance clustering of rare events. It is easier to see the effects of a teratogen in a maternity hospital, with between 2000 and 6000 births a year. However, if only a low proportion of women or their partners are exposed to the teratogen, the numbers of babies affected will still be small and again may be ascribed to chance. It is not until figures on malformations from hundreds of thousands of pregnancies are aggregated that the effects of health hazards can be shown with any degree of certainty. This can be done through the use of congenital malformation and genetic registers.

Registers use information from individuals as part of good epidemiological studies. These may lead to the formation of hypotheses as to the cause of malformations in populations which can be tested scientifically. This may suggest ways of detecting the malformation through screening individuals in that population who have the characteristics that make that malformation more likely to happen (the high risk population).

Examples of the use of epidemiology that have resulted in finding the causes of malformations include the effects of thalidomide on limb formation in fetuses, the effects of maternal rubella and the increased incidence of malformations in women on insulin who have poorly controlled diabetes at the time of conception.

ASSESSING THE NEED FOR SCREENING

There is always a risk that any plans to implement screening for congenital malformations and disorders may be seen as a 'search and destroy mission' by public health specialists, sacrificing individuals with a problem for the greater good of society – the utilitarian approach mentioned in the chapter on ethics.

Resources for health care are finite and so purchasers of health care have a 'portfolio' of services that they buy. This usually means buying a little of everything rather than excellent health care for only one section of society. Purchasers need to buy cost-effective health care which provides good outcomes for the public money spent on them. However, there are definite problems of the use of cost-effectiveness analysis in looking at prenatal screening. It might be taken to imply that terminating an abnormal pregnancy saves the state from having to pay for expensive lifelong health care for a disabled person and so money spent on screening is well spent as it means money is saved on health care elsewhere. However, this implies that screening should only be offered when parents agree to have a termination if there is an abnormality. Naturally, this view disturbs those with malformations, as it begins to suggest that health care for any particular disorder may not be provided by a state-funded health service if that disorder can be detected prenatally.

One of the main values put on prenatal screening and diagnosis is the information that it yields to individuals to enable parents to make informed choices about their situation. It is impossible to put a monetary value on the benefit of information to include in a cost/benefit analysis.

Technology exists to screen and diagnose several hundred genetic disorders and many of the population will want to take advantage of new tests. Public health can contribute to the debate about what tests should be available by using epidemiology to look at and assess the need for screening services – what are the commonest genetic disorders in the local population, what are the areas where intervention could reduce the burden of disease by preventing further disability ?

EVALUATING PILOT SCREENING PROJECTS

Screening is a service that detects the predisposition for a particular disease or its early, treatable stages in people who are generally considered to be disease-free when the screen is carried out. Public health evaluates how well screening tests perform in picking up individuals who will develop disease.

A screening test is not usually in itself diagnostic; it detects a subgroup of those tested who are at higher risk of having the disease or disorder than the original population screened. This subgroup needs further investigation with a diagnostic test which is often more time-consuming, expensive and invasive than the screening test. For example, the questions 'How old are you?' and 'What ethnic group do you belong to?' are both screening tests to determine a subgroup which is at higher risk of having a baby with a problem than the general population – trisomy 21 in the case of maternal age, and sickle cell anaemia, thalassaemia or Tay–Sachs disease in the case of ethnic group. Further investigation in the form of a diagnostic amniocentesis or a blood test to pick up sickle cell trait are needed to confirm or refute that the condition is present. Once the diagnosis is confirmed, treatment or preventive advice and action can be offered. This in itself creates conflicts – public health can supply figures on the risks of having a baby with an abnormality on which to base informed consent, but if you are the one individual in 1000 who is considered to be at high risk, that is 100% of you.

Public health practitioners have a duty to the general population to ensure that any screening programme is effective – that it picks up individuals who are truly at high risk and offers them further diagnostic tests, and does not reassure parents that they are at low risk and then confront them with a handicapped baby because the low risk was wrongly assessed.

A screening test may be read as negative even if the disease is present (a false negative), thus giving both the person screened and their medical advisors false reassurance that all is well. It may, on the other hand, be read as positive when a disease is not present (a false positive), which will lead to further unnecessary investigation before the actual health of the person screened is confirmed. These errors occur because most screening tests are not discrete and do not measure the absolute presence or absence of disease. Instead, they measure biochemical parameters of a disorder. For example, serum alpha fetoprotein is found in maternal serum in all pregnancies; an arbitrary cut-off point for high and low values at different gestational ages is needed to use the value of serum alpha fetoprotein as a screening test for open neural tube defects and for chromosomal abnormalities. The efficacy of the programme in picking up a high proportion of true cases without subjecting hundreds of pregnancies to the potential dangers of an invasive diagnostic test, such as amniocentesis, with all the dilemmas which it involves, needs a careful balance of risks.

If a screening programme is to be assessed for its effectiveness, two questions need to be asked.

1. **To what extent can the test discriminate between affected and unaffected individuals?**

   There are two measures to assess the discriminatory powers of a screening programme. The first is the **specificity** – the proportion of unaffected individuals who have a negative result on screening. An example of this is the proportion of women who have normal babies who get a negative result (low or normal AFP) from a serum screen for neural tube defect.

   The second is called the **sensitivity** of a screening programme. It is the proportion of affected individuals who give a positive result on screening and is also known as the detection rate of the programme. An example is the proportion of women who have babies with a neural tube defect who will be found to have a positive result (high AFP) on a serum screen for neural tube defect.

2. **What is the chance that those who have a positive screening test really have the disease?**

   This is a measure of the proportion of true positive screening tests to all positive screening tests and is known as the **predictive value**. The sensitivity and specificity of a screen remain the same, however many cases there are in a population. In contrast, the predictive value depends on the prevalence of the disorder in the population screened. If tests are introduced in populations where there is a high prevalence of the disease (for example, relatives of people with inherited disorders), the odds of being affected may be high and a screening test will pick up many cases. However, the screening test will be less impressive in the general population where the prevalence of the disorder is lower.

Screening programmes are offered routinely to all members of the population included in the programme as a target group, for example, all women over 37 years of age. As this target population consists of people who are healthy, it is extremely important that the advantages of testing for the disorder should not be outweighed by the disadvantages. Screening may be more effective if it is targeted to an identifiable high risk group rather than attempting to cover the whole population. People known to be at high risk of genetic disease because a member of their family has developed the illness are usually counselled about their risks and are aware of the possibilities of prenatal diagnosis. They are therefore more likely to comply with a screening procedure than people who are suddenly offered a test to pick up a disease of which they have never heard and which they have never considered might cause problems for them. However, most recessive disorders (such as cystic fibrosis) occur in couples with no family history because of the nature of the 1 in 4 risk of inheritance. Individuals might rightly be angry if they were not targeted for a simple carrier screening test which would have highlighted their high risk because the problem had not manifested itself in their family.

Public health practitioners also have a duty to ensure that services are given to each person efficiently – that is, that the input of resources into screening programmes produces the maximum output in the form of information that can be used by couples to give informed consent to procedures. Screening has been applied to a variety of diseases with no simple genetic origins (for example hypertension, cervical cancer, urine dip stick testing for diabetes and proteinuria are all screened for during pregnancy) with a wide variety of success in achieving the primary aim of screening – to prevent morbidity and mortality from the disease (Mant and Fowler, 1990). Lessons can be learnt from screening programmes applied to these diseases. These include how to educate health care professionals and those in the target group about the screen and how to feed back the results of the screen (whether positive or negative) so that diagnostic tests, treatment or preventive measures can be offered. Education of both professionals and public is essential if the screening test is to be offered and taken up by the whole of the target population. The full potential benefits of a programme can only be realized if a large proportion of the target group voluntarily attends for screening.

The term 'disease state' differentiates genetic from other forms of screening. Screening programmes are usually designed to benefit the individual tested directly, by offering either early diagnosis and treatment or prevention or by reassurance that there is one less disease the person tested currently has to worry about. There is no direct benefit to individuals tested in a genetic screening programme from knowing their genetic carrier status other than allowing them to make choices about their future family. Carrier status does **not** mean that the carrier of a recessive disorder is diseased, as their other 'normal' gene will compensate for the presence of the abnormal one. However, without such screening, definitive prenatal diagnostic tests cannot be offered.

There is a very real danger that genetic screening may lead to the perception that carriers are abnormal and diseased. In 1974 in Seattle, Hampton and colleagues showed that hastily introduced screening programmes led to sickle cell 'non-disease' with carrier children being regarded as 'different' by parents. There are also dangers that carriers may be disadvantaged when applying for health insurance – will a private company insure a couple with a one in four risk of having a child with cystic fibrosis unless they undertake to terminate any affected pregnancy?

As the genes that cause disease are mapped and cloned, it will become more common to perform a screening test that is also diagnostic in that it detects the actual presence of a gene mutation causing a disease rather than a biochemical test which detects and measures the gene product. Genetic screening is therefore starting to differ from most other forms of screening in that it is the final arbiter of whether the person tested is positive or negative for the 'disease state' or presence of the gene. The possibility of screening for carriers of cystic fibrosis was raised by the identification, in 1990, of a three base-pair deletion (delta F508) in the structural gene for cystic fibrosis on the long arm of chromosome seven (Rommens *et al.*, 1990). The realization of the technical feasibility of cystic fibrosis carrier screening by detecting the faulty gene itself has produced strong arguments both for and against its introduction. (Modell, 1990; Wilfond and Fost, 1990)

The greatest difference between screening for genetic diseases and for other disorders is that true primary prevention is not currently possible for genetic disorders. There are several options open to carriers of an inherited disease to avoid the birth of an affected child, but many of these are not generally acceptable to individuals or couples:

- to remain childless, whether by remaining single or by voluntarily foregoing the opportunity to have children;
- to select a partner who is not a carrier of the same disease;
- to use artificial insemination by donor or another form of assisted reproduction;
- ensuring that only a non-affected fetus implants by preimplantation diagnosis on an eight-cell embryo (Coutelle *et al.*, 1989; Handyside *et al.*, 1992);
- to terminate a pregnancy found by antenatal diagnosis to be affected.

Recent advances in the field of gene and cell transplantation (Editorial 1990a) may offer true hope of secondary prevention and increase the acceptability of genetic screening programmes. However, the spectre of eugenic control of future generations hangs over genetic screening programmes and the issue needs to be addressed if they are to succeed and lay the foundations for future programmes when true prevention is a viable option.

Given that primary prevention is not a current possibility, the objectives of genetic screening developed by the Royal College of Physicians of London (1989) are different from those of other screening programmes. They are:

- to allow the widest possible range of informed choice to women and couples at risk of having children with an abnormality;
- to provide reassurance and reduce the level of anxiety associated with reproduction;
- to allow couples to embark on having a family knowing that they may avoid the birth of seriously affected children through selective abortion;
- to ensure optimal treatment of affected infants through early diagnosis.

There are many different screening programmes for many different types of disease. Various sets of criteria by which to judge whether a screening programme is likely to bring benefits to those screened have been published (Thorner and Remein, 1961; McKeown, 1968; Cochrane and Holland, 1971; Wilson and Junger, 1968; Cuckle and Wald, 1984).

To summarize the criteria for a successful screening programme, the genetic disorder which is being sought by the programme should:

- be well defined;
- be of known natural history;
- be an important health problem for the individual and for the community as it is severe, or common or both;
- be of known incidence and prevalence;
- be preventable by acceptable methods;
- have a beneficial influence on reproductive decision making by detection of carrier status.

The screening test must be:

- simple, safe and acceptable;
- valid, that is both sensitive and specific with a high predictive value;
- repeatable;
- relatively inexpensive.

Moreover, the distribution of test values in affected and unaffected individuals must be known, a suitable cut-off level defined and the extent of overlap must be sufficiently small.

As screening tests are applied to people who are regarded as being fit and well in an attempt to stop future ill health, it is vital that tests are acceptable and do not cause iatrogenic disease. Acceptability varies according to culture and perceived seriousness of the disorder – it is accepted in western countries that women should not mind having a vaginal examination with a speculum in order for a cervical smear to be taken because it is perceived that the screening procedure will have a significant effect on mortality from cervical cancer.

In any screening programme, it is inevitable that certain individuals will be subject to what is later proved to be unnecessary worry and that some will be falsely reassured and thus be even more devastated by the birth of a child with a congenital malformation. Evaluation of screening programmes is therefore essential if individuals in society are to have access to appropriate technology which overall does more good than harm.

INFORMING PUBLIC POLICY DECISIONS ABOUT SCREENING

Costs of medical care are rising worldwide and the premise on which the British National Health Service was founded – if money is spent on health care, then the need for health care systems to treat disease will reduce over a period of time – has been shown to be wrong time and again. Better health services bring higher expectations in the population funding the service through taxes or insurance contributions and increase demand for care. Steep rises in spending on health care have led to the introduction of cash limits to nationalized health care services and limits as to what insurers would pay in private health care systems. Those funding health care are concerned about value for the money they spend and this has led to the need to show that clinical practice in obstetrics is safe and effective. Failure of free markets for health care and equal access to care for all citizens are the reasons why in all countries the state has a role in preventive and curative health services.

Issues such as these are now an integral part of the debate between politicians, health managers and the public before change in maternity services can occur. In reality, this involves an ongoing dialogue between parents represented by pressure groups, health care professionals and politicians, none of whom can claim an exclusive right to give the final solution. There is a conflict between the personal, family view of giving birth as an important physiological life event versus the requirements of politicians, tax payers, insurance companies and professionals for safety and value for money. In our present day egalitarian society, public debate is regarded as entirely acceptable but there are undoubtedly drawbacks in compromise solutions which attempt to satisfy all parties.

The arrival of technology as an established part of care in pregnancy, while solving many problems, has also introduced new ones. The pregnant woman and her obstetrician no longer wait for delivery accepting that whatever happens is 'God's will'. The woman expects that those who care for her have access to the latest technology for the care of her and her baby and that she will be kept fully informed of the implications of using that technology and any abnormal findings.

Screening tests for fetal wellbeing are now used in all maternity units. These range from methods for detecting fetal abnormality to biophysical and biochemical assessment of the fetus. Clinical decision making is very dependent on such tests – for example, whether or not to terminate a pregnancy when a fetal anomaly is suspected. Recently Chalmers and colleagues (1989) have drawn attention to the considerable variation in the validity of some of these tests and interventions. Routine ultrasound screening for fetal anomaly has never been subjected to a scientific evaluation in the form of a randomized controlled trial. However, its use in the United Kingdom is now so widespread that it now might be considered unethical not to offer an anomaly scan to one group in a randomized controlled trial. The situation appears to be different in the United States, where scanning has not taken hold to the extent it has done in the United Kingdom. Provision of scanning as a routine has been driven by clinicians who want to detect abnormality and parents who want the chance to see and welcome their baby in the womb and confirm their child's normality. Tensions arise because the aims of these two groups are actually at odds with each other.

If care is to be evaluated scientifically, women and their partners have to understand the basis of randomized trials and agree to take part in the studies needed. Unless women agree to be allocated by drawing numbers to specific treatment or non-treatment groups, professionals cannot give future mothers the benefit of proper information on which to base their choices. Many women are altruistic enough to agree to take part in trials where they cannot see any particular advantage or disadvantage to being in one or other group – however, unless trials take place soon after the introduction of a new technique or technology, women can be as blinded by the perceived but anecdotal and unquantified advantages or disadvantages as their doctors.

Health care professionals treat individuals, but treating an individual may produce other consequences which affect third parties – for example, immunizing a person against rubella makes them less likely to pass the disease on to women who may be pregnant as well as giving individual protection (Normand, 1991). Many people pay for their own health care through insurance or directly from their own pockets, but a considerable amount of care is paid for by the state in most western countries through taxation. The consequence of this is that benefits produced for one section of the community may mean that resources are not available for care which would benefit another section. Similarly, screening programmes which would benefit individuals directly may not be initiated if the results are not important for the community as a whole. An example of this is screening for toxoplasmosis in pregnancy.

The parasite *Toxoplasma gondii* can cause fetal infection resulting in severe and lasting neurological damage in the baby when the mother contracts the infection for the first time in pregnancy. The disease in the mother is usually symptomless and not all infections in pregnancy produce disability in the baby. Screening programmes on maternal blood have been running in France and Austria for some time. An initial test is done at booking and, if the mother has not had a previous *Toxoplasma* infection, the tests are repeated monthly to ensure that any new infection is detected and treated *in utero* and a termination of pregnancy is offered if necessary. About 20–25% of French women need repeated testing (Editorial, 1990b)

In Britain, about 25 new cases of congenital toxoplasmosis are reported each year to the British Paediatric Surveillance Unit in 680 000 births. This is about half the expected number estimated from data on acute *Toxoplasma* infection in pregnancy and transmission rates (Editorial, 1990b). Only 20% of women tested in London had previously had a toxoplasmosis infection (Fleck, 1969), so a screening programme in the United Kingdom would need to test 680 000 women at the start of their pregnancy and subsequently 80% or 540 000 pregnant women in each month of their pregnancy to produce the chance of detecting 25–50 cases each year. The expense of this means that it is highly unlikely that toxoplasmosis screening will be introduced in Britain. This is in spite of vigorous lobbying by well-informed and highly motivated pressure groups of families who have discovered that their child has been damaged by a potentially detectable and treatable disease. The cost per case discovered, however beneficial to the individual family concerned, is simply too high. Greater benefit to the community as a whole might result from spending the same amount of money on other forms of more cost-beneficial health care. Health education about minimizing the risks of contracting toxoplasmosis during pregnancy through food hygiene in preparing raw meat and in avoiding cat faeces is a more cost-effective way of reducing the incidence. (Royal College of Obstetricians and Gynaecologists Multidisciplinary Working Group, 1992)

A similar dilemma arises with serum screening for the chromosomal defect trisomy 21 (Down syndrome). Current screening programmes based on offering amniocentesis to older mothers (37 years old or more) subject about 5% of pregnancies in Britain to amniocentesis and pick up about one third of fetuses with trisomy 21. Newer techniques, using markers found in maternal blood, have been shown to pick up nearly half of all cases for the same amniocentesis rate. (Wald *et al.*, 1992) However, to keep to the same 5% amniocentesis rate, older mothers will have to forego their absolute right to a diagnostic test and will only have an amniocentesis if indicated by the blood test, which misses one-third of cases. Some sort of cost/benefit evaluation is needed for all screening programmes, together with surveys on what those who are most affected by the results, the parents, think of what is offered to them.

MONITORING THE RESULTS OF POPULATION SCREENING PROGRAMMES

Research is done by interested and enthusiastic clinicians who are motivated to produce successful findings that have an effect on everyday clinical practice. However, there is a development phase in promulgating research findings to units who have not developed the techniques required along with the research. An example of this is the Medical Research Council trial of amniocentesis (1978), which found that miscarriage directly related to amniocentesis occurred in 1–1.5% of pregnancies tested in this way. This rate is commonly quoted to parents, but the outcome is also related to the experience of the operator – if more than two insertions are made during any one procedure, the fetal loss rate is increased (Simpson *et al.*, 1976; Lowe *et al.*, 1978). Thus parents should ask 'What are the risks of a miscarriage if you or a member of your team do my amniocentesis' and not 'What are the risks of an amniocentesis causing a miscarriage?'. Audit is the term applied to a systematic review of how a technique proved by research to produce good patient care is applied in practice. In local units, clinicians have a duty to audit their own practice to identify areas where they could improve and to ensure that specified standards of care are achieved. Public health and purchasers have a duty to ensure that audit takes place and that clinical areas where problems have been identified are audited and changes to improve care are implemented.

Not all research findings can be translated directly into programmes that produce health gain predicted from the research. Retrospective analysis of stored serum from pregnancies which resulted in a fetus with trisomy 21 (Wald, Cuckle and Densem, 1988) suggested that two-thirds of cases could be picked up for a 5% false positive rate. In practice (Wald *et al.*, 1992) just over half the cases were picked up in a demonstration project, largely because take-up of screening varied considerably. If the public votes with its feet and does not take up screening programmes, their effectiveness decreases and tough decisions have to be made as to whether to divert more resources into promoting the programme or to stop the programme altogether. In practice, this rarely happens and several screening programmes have outlived their usefulness – for example, even when the incidence of tuberculosis fell and treatment with antibiotics became effective, it took some time before mass miniature X-ray population screening was abandoned. Pressure on health service budgets means that public health has a vital role in monitoring screening programmes to ensure that they are, and remain, effective in reaching their goals – a form of large scale audit.

Starting and stopping screening entails considerable debate and must be done on good evidence of efficacy and efficiency rather than anecdotes. The practice of good public health can raise the standard of this debate and can ensure that the conflicts engendered in preventing disease, prolonging life and promoting health for the individual through using the efforts and resources produced by society in an organized way are addressed.

REFERENCES

Acheson, D. (1988) Public health in England – the report of the committee of enquiry into the future development of the public health function, *Cmd 289*, HMSO, London.

Chalmers, I., Enkin, M.W. and Kierse, M.J.N.C. (eds) (1989) *Effective Care in Pregnancy and Childbirth*, Oxford University Press, Oxford.

Cochrane, A.L. and Holland, W.W. (1971) Validation of screening procedures. *British Medical Bulletin*, **27**, 3.

Coutelle, C., Williams, C., Handyside, A. *et al.* (1989) Genetic analysis of DNA from single human oocytes: a model for preimplantation diagnosis of cystic fibrosis. *British Medical Journal*, **299**, 22–24.

Cuckle, H.S. and Wald, N.J. (1984) Principles of screening, in *Antenatal and Neonatal Screening*, (ed. N.J. Wald), Oxford University Press, Oxford, pp. 1–21.

Editorial (1990a) Myoblast transfer in Duchenne's muscular dystrophy. *British Medical Journal*, **301**, 77–78

Editorial (1990b) Antenatal screening for toxoplasmosis in the United Kingdom. *Lancet*, **ii**, 346–347

Fleck, D.G. (1969) Toxoplasmosis. *Public Health*, **83**, 131–135.

Hampton, M.L., Anderson, J., Lavizzo, B.S. *et al.* (1974) Sickle cell 'non-disease', a potentially serious public health problem. *American Journal of Diseases of Childhood*, **128**, 58–61.

Handyside, A.H., Lesko, J.G., Tarin, J.J. *et al.* (1992). Birth of a normal girl after *in vitro* fertilisation and preimplantation diagnostic testing for cystic fibrosis. *New England Journal of Medicine*, **327**, 905–909.

Lowe, C.U., Alexander, D., Bryla, D. *et al.* (1978) *The Safety and Accuracy of Mid-trimester Amniocentesis*, US Department of Health, Education and Welfare DHEW Publication number (NIH) 78-190, DHEW, Washington, DC.

McKeown, T. (1968) Validation of screening procedures, in *Screening in Medical Care. Reviewing the Evidence* (Nuffield Provincial Hospital Trust), Oxford University Press, Oxford.

Mant, D. and Fowler, G. (1990) Mass screening: theory and ethics. *British Medical Journal*, **300**, 916–918.

Medical Research Council (1978) An assessment of the hazards of amniocentesis. *British Journal of Obstetrics and Gynaecology*, **85**(suppl 2), 1–41.

Modell, B. (1990). Cystic fibrosis screening and community genetics. *Journal of Medical Genetics*, **27**, 475–479.

Mooney, G. (1992) *Economics, Medicine and Health Care*, 2nd edn, Harvester Wheatsheaf, Hemel Hempstead, Bucks.

Normand, C. (1991) Economics, health, and the economics of health. *British Medical Journal*, **303**, 1572–1577.

Rommens, J.M., Ianuzzi, M.C., Kerem B-S. *et al.* (1990) Identification of the cystic fibrosis gene: chromosome walking and jumping. *Science*, **245**, 1059–1065.

Royal College of Obstetricians and Gynaecologists Multidisciplinary Working Group (1992) *Prenatal Screening for Toxoplasmosis in the United Kingdom*, Royal College of Obstetricians and Gynaecologists, London.

Royal College of Physicians of London (1989) *Prenatal Diagnosis and Screening – Community and Service Implications*, Royal College of Physicians, London.

Simpson, N.E., Dallaire, L., Miller, J.R. *et al.* (1976) Prenatal diagnosis of genetic disease in Canada: report of a collaborative study. *Canadian Medical Association Journal*, **115**, 739–746.

Thorner, R.M. and Remein, Q.R. (1961) *Principles and Procedures in the Evaluation of Screening for Disease*, Public Health Monograph 67. US Department of Health Education and Welfare, Washington, DC.

Wald, N.J., Cuckle, H.S. and Densem, J.W. (1988) Maternal serum screening for Down syndrome in early pregnancy. *British Medical Journal*, **297**, 883–887.

Wald, N.J., Kennard, A., Densem, J.W. *et al.* (1992) Antenatal maternal serum screening for Down's syndrome: results of a demonstration project. *British Medical Journal*, **305**, 391–394.

Wilfond, B.S. and Fost, N. (1990) The cystic fibrosis gene; medical and social implications for heterozygote detection. *Journal of the American Medical Association*, **263**, 2777–2783.

Wilson, J.M.C. and Junger, G. (1968) *Principles and Practice of Screening for Disease*, WHO Public Health Papers 34, World Health Organization, Geneva.

5

Counselling prior to prenatal testing

Lenore Abramsky

Should women be counselled prior to having prenatal diagnostic tests? If so, why, how, where and by whom? What constitutes a prenatal diagnostic test? This chapter will consider all these issues and explore some of the dilemmas created by the new technology. The first dilemma is how to refer to the counsellor who, because of the constraints of the English language, must be assigned a gender. I have decided to give her my own. The term 'counsellor' will be used to refer to anyone doing counselling, whatever the actual training or qualifications of that person may be.

WHY COUNSEL?

Why is it more important to counsel a woman before taking her blood for alpha fetoprotein than it is to counsel her prior to taking blood to see if she is anaemic? What is the essential difference between these two tests? The difference lies in the purpose for which the tests are done.

Taking the mother's blood to see if she is anaemic is done in order to safeguard the health of the mother and therefore of the baby. If the mother is anaemic, she can be given iron supplementation. For the majority of women in western countries, this remedy will be acceptable. The implied value judgement expressed in doing this test and acting upon it is that it is a good thing if both mother and baby are kept as healthy as possible. Most women would concur with this value judgement unless it involves what for them is an unacceptable amount of interference in their lives or in the pregnancy.

The purpose of prenatal diagnostic tests is, for the most part, quite different. They are done so that if the baby is affected with a serious handicap the parents can choose to have the pregnancy terminated if they wish (Crawfurd, 1983). The implied value judgement expressed in doing these tests is that if the quality of life will not be good enough (which is open to interpretation) then it is preferable that there be no life. Many people, but by no means everyone, would agree with this statement. The counsellor who says 'we recommend an amniocentesis for all women your age' rather than 'we offer an amniocentesis for all woman your age' is assuming that the woman does agree with the statement and is putting subtle pressure on her to have the test. For those who do not agree that no life is preferable to 'poor-quality life' it is far from clear that it is always beneficial for them to know early in pregnancy that the baby will be born with a serious handicap. I have certainly been told by some people that they would rather not have known about the handicap before the baby was born while others are very grateful that they did know.

Another complication is that some prenatal diagnostic tests are invasive and carry with them a risk to the pregnancy (Turnbull and MacKenzie, 1983; Rodeck and Nicolaides, 1983; Canadian Collaborative CVS-Amniocentesis Clinical Trial Group, 1989; MRC Working Party on the Evaluation of Chorion Villus Sampling, 1991). No parents should be asked to take that risk unless they fully understand it and are entirely sure that the information to be obtained is worth the risk they would be taking.

The qualitative difference between the purpose of prenatal diagnostic tests and most other medical tests might be better understood by looking at an analogous situation that does not involve pregnancy.

If a person goes to his general practitioner for a check-up, the doctor is probably safe in assuming that the patient would like to have a blood test to check for anaemia, so that treatment can be initiated if the patient is anaemic. By virtue of being there, the patient has expressed an interest in maintaining his health. It would be a very different story if the doctor were doing the blood test not in order to treat any abnormality found but with a view to offering the patient euthanasia if the result were abnormal. If this were the purpose of the test, the doctor would not be correct in assuming that the patient wanted the test just because he was there, and it would be necessary to counsel him and to obtain informed consent before doing any tests. In the same way, the doctor or midwife in the antenatal clinic or the genetics clinic cannot assume that just because a woman is there she wants prenatal diagnostic tests with the possible consequence of being offered a termination of pregnancy.

WHAT CONSTITUTES A PRENATAL DIAGNOSTIC TEST?

If it is accepted that counselling is appropriate before prenatal screening and diagnostic tests are done, the next issue is to identify which investigations are prenatal diagnostic tests. We would probably all agree that amniocentesis, chorionic villus sampling and fetal blood sampling are prenatal diagnostic tests. Most people would agree that serum screening (whether it be alpha fetoprotein only or one of the combined methods) is part of a process in prenatal diagnosis. Many people are not, however, fully aware that ultrasound scanning is our most powerful tool in the field of prenatal diagnosis in that it is the investigation offered to the most women and the one which detects the most fetal abnormalities (Chitty *et al.*, 1991; Levi *et al.*, 1991; Shirley, Bottomley and Robinson, 1992).

The more physically invasive the test is, the more risk it poses to the pregnancy and the more counselling the woman gets prior to the test. So a woman might have much counselling prior to a fetal blood sampling and absolutely no counselling prior to an ultrasound scan. This takes into account the woman's right to decide whether or not to expose the pregnancy to risk but ignores her right to decide whether or not she wants to have certain information about her baby.

WHAT CONSTITUTES ADEQUATE PRE-TEST COUNSELLING?

The next issue for consideration is what the purposes of the counselling are and what constitutes adequate counselling. These questions have been considered by others and are discussed by Green (1990). In my view, pre-test counselling must ensure firstly that the woman is adequately informed about the condition being tested for and knows as much as possible about the test being offered so that she and her partner can make a fully informed decision about whether or not to have it. This means she needs to know what her own prior risk (without the benefit of the test results) is for the condition to be tested and this risk should be put in context. She must also know what that condition is. She needs to know how, where and when the test would be done, what it would feel like and what aftercare might be needed. She must be clear about whether it is a screening test or a diagnostic test and how accurate it is for a person in her situation. She needs information about what sorts of condition could be screened for or diagnosed and what sorts of condition could not be detected by the test in question. She needs to be aware of the risks involved to the pregnancy and the possible consequences of receiving the information the test provides. She should also be aware of what alternative tests are available to look for the same condition. It will be seen that this is a very long list of information necessary if the woman is to be fully informed. This amount of information cannot be imparted without some time being spent. It also cannot be imparted by staff who are not fully informed themselves. Such a large amount of information is unlikely to be remembered accurately by most people. For this reason, it should be backed up with clear written material.

It is worth noting here that even among women who state at the outset of counselling that they have already made up their minds about what they will do, some change their minds when they become better informed about the tests (Abramsky and Rodeck, 1991). Three pieces of information which women tend to cite as reasons for changing their minds about tests are:

- the level of risk they have for the condition in question;
- the miscarriage risk of the test being considered;
- the method of termination which would be offered if they chose to terminate the pregnancy following an abnormal result from the test in question.

The second purpose of pre-test counselling is to help those women or couples who are having trouble making a decision to reach a decision which is suitable for them. Essentially, the role of the counsellor is to help the woman or couple to see what all the possible consequences of having or not having the tests in question would be and to determine which set of consequences is the most acceptable (or the least unacceptable) to her or them.

This requires more time, skill and sensitivity on the part of the counsellor, and very definitely does not involve counsellors giving advice which is essentially what they think they would do in the situation. What the counsellors would do is entirely irrelevant. It is not their baby and they will not have to live with the consequences of any decisions which are made. It is important to help the counsellee to explore the pros and cons for her of having the test in question, a different test or no test. Many people are helped in this by a 'worst scenario exercise' (Lippman-Hand and Fraser, 1979). They may, for example, want to consider whether to them the miscarriage of a healthy baby would be worse than, or less or equally as bad as, the birth of a handicapped child. With the 'worst case scenario' it is necessary for the couple to keep in mind the relative likelihood of the various end results. If handled well, this exercise can help a lot of people to come to a decision which is right for them.

CAN PRE-TEST COUNSELLING BE NON-DIRECTIVE?

I have argued that pre-test counselling should be non-directive since it is the counsellee and not the counsellor whose entire future life may be affected by decisions made at the session. However, we must ask whether non-directive pre-test counselling is achievable. Powerful arguments have been made that it is not possible (Clarke, 1991). Those present at the Third European Meeting on Psychosocial Aspects of Genetics (1992) voted by a narrow majority that non-directive genetic counselling was not achievable in practice. This is partly because the counsellor comes to the session with her own cultural background, personality and life experiences. She probably has her own views about what she thinks she would do in the situation or what she thinks a responsible person should do. These views may be conscious or unconscious but they will influence her choice of words in describing conditions, tests and probabilities. They will influence her facial expression and body language, the order in which things are explained and the amount of time spent on different topics. The good counsellor will do her best to understand her own feelings and to try to keep them out of the counselling situation, but this may not always be entirely successful.

The second stumbling block making non-directive counselling difficult to achieve in the antenatal context is the fact that most women having prenatal tests do not approach someone asking for them; they are offered such tests as routine anomaly scanning, amniocentesis for advanced maternal age, serum screening for neural tube defects or Down syndrome, carrier testing for thalassaemia, sickle cell disease, Tay–Sachs disease or cystic fibrosis. When we offer such tests, are we not saying that the condition being tested for is undesirable and that we are offering the patient/client the opportunity of knowing about it in time to end the pregnancy if the baby is affected? We therefore start many counselling sessions in a way which suggests a possible direction. Many women find it difficult to refuse a test which has been offered (Sjogren and Uddenberg, 1988). However, we have an unsolvable problem. If we do not offer the tests, then the only people to have access to prenatal diagnosis will be well-informed women who ask for it, and this is clearly unjust.

It seems that we cannot offer tests without being somewhat directive; we must therefore be extremely careful in both what we say and what written information is given out to explain to people the optional nature of these tests and the fact that it is entirely acceptable to decline the offer. We must be certain to say that we 'offer' all women (or all those in a given category) the test but not say that we 'advise' them to have it.

HOW IS PRE-TEST COUNSELLING DONE IN PRACTICE?

We have considered some of the reasons why informative, sensitive, non-directive counselling is desirable prior to a woman embarking upon prenatal diagnostic tests. It is important to set high standards in this area, but it is equally important to live in the real world with our feet on the ground and to see how things are, in fact, done and what practical steps can be taken to bridge the inevitable gap between the actual and the ideal.

Pre-test counselling probably comes closest to the ideal in the context of the genetics services. In such services couples are counselled by clinical geneticists and specialist genetic counsellors who are likely to have up-to-date information, to understand what it means, to be skilled in explaining it and to have the necessary aids such as pictures and diagrams. They are also experienced at this particular type of counselling. In addition, the time allowed for such discussion in the genetics services is far greater than that allowed in most antenatal clinics and there is often a greater degree of privacy.

Perhaps most importantly, the ethos of genetic counselling has traditionally been such that the counsellor provides information so that the counsellee can make informed choices (Harper, 1981). This contrasts sharply with the practice in most other fields of medicine in which both doctors and nurses may be used to telling patients what they should do.

It is extremely difficult for someone who has offered directive counselling for years to become non-directive for particular occasions. So it is not surprising that in the context of ordinary antenatal care, tests are often presented as routine rather than as one possible course of action. In one study (Marteau *et al.* 1992) looking at counselling prior to serum alpha fetoprotein tests, it was found that over half the doctors presented it as routine, saying things such as 'and also we do a routine blood test for spina bifida', and did not invite the woman to make a decision. This is even more true of anomaly scanning, which in the United Kingdom tends to be presented as routine care with no discussion about the possibility of finding abnormalities or about whether the woman would like to have it done. Literature given to women may say that the scan is 'to make sure that the baby is developing normally'. One well-used leaflet, referring to urine and blood tests and scans, said 'the previous tests are the routine ones carried out on all pregnant women'.

It is not possible or desirable for all pregnant women to have full-scale genetic counselling, so the vast majority of women will continue to receive what pre-test counselling they get from those looking after them in the course of their routine antenatal care. With this in mind, I decided to look at the professed practices in one health region with regard to amniocentesis counselling for advanced maternal age.

A questionnaire about counselling before amniocentesis was sent to all maternity units in one health region in England. Completed questionnaires were returned from all units giving a general picture about professed counselling practices in the region.

It emerged that in the typical unit, women were counselled by a senior doctor or a midwife during a routine antenatal visit and that such counselling lasted between 5 and 15 minutes.

There were only two pieces of information which counsellors from all units said they gave; they were the woman's age-specific risk for Down syndrome and the risk that an amniocentesis would cause a miscarriage.

Counsellors from roughly two-thirds of the units said that they also told women about the conditions which could not be identified by amniocentesis, what the amniocentesis felt like, what the recommended aftercare was and what alternative tests were available.

Counsellors from fewer than half the units said that they mentioned the culture failure rate after amniocentesis or explained what a mid-trimester termination involved. It could be argued that any woman who consents to an amniocentesis without knowing what sort of termination she would be offered in the event of an abnormal result has not given informed consent to the procedure. She is not aware of a very basic possible consequence of the investigation.

Finally, in fewer than one-third of the units were the possibility of a false negative on amniocentesis or the age risk for chromosome abnormalities other than Down syndrome mentioned. This last omission is particularly important if one considers that up to half the chromosome abnormalities picked up on amniocentesis may not be Down syndrome (Ferguson-Smith, 1983). If a couple have embarked upon amniocentesis thinking that Down syndrome is the only condition which might be diagnosed and that they would definitely terminate in such an event, they are likely to react to all abnormalities with a knee jerk reaction of 'terminate'. If the result is an abnormality such as Klinefelter syndrome, the parents who are not aware of such a possibility may close their minds to any information about the condition because they 'know that they want a termination'. Parents may also, in the words of Barbara Katz Rothman (1986) find themselves 'incapacitated by this information, ...incapable of mothering [the child]'.

Staff from just over half the units said that they gave out detailed written information about amniocentesis. They supplied copies of the leaflets used. The quality of the leaflets varied enormously. At one end there were well-written, clear, informative handouts. At the other there were poorly written, unclear, out of date, inaccurate leaflets.

Compare, for example, the following extracts about possible pregnancy termination from two very different leaflets:

> If the results show that your baby is handicapped, the doctor will discuss the options with you and your partner. They will offer to terminate the pregnancy.... You may, however, decide to keep the baby and take advantage of the time to prepare for the care of your child.

> The only treatment for babies with a serious congenital abnormality is termination of pregnancy.

Look at the difference between these two descriptions of ultrasound anomaly scanning taken from different leaflets:

> Ultrasound can also be used to look for certain abnormalities such as spina bifida. It cannot detect everything, however, and some problems may be missed.

> This [the 19-week scan] is done to check that the baby has no abnormalities that cannot be detected by the ultrasound at 15–16 weeks, as it was too early to do this.

Some leaflets stressed the optional nature of the tests, for example:

> Please note that the test is offered to you, but the decision as to whether you wish it to be done is yours. You may feel that if you are carrying a baby with Down syndrome, you wish to continue with the pregnancy; that choice is also yours.

Other leaflets made no explicit mention of the optional nature of amniocentesis.

It is worth noting that no-one sent in examples of leaflets in any language other than English, and only one respondent spontaneously mentioned that they had such leaflets. It is possible that more units had material in other languages, as this question was not specifically asked. If written information is available only in English, there will be many women for whom no written information is available.

WHAT DO WOMEN SAY THEY WANT FROM PRE-TEST COUNSELLING?

I also asked a series of women attending for advanced maternal age counselling at one of the hospitals surveyed to write about what they hoped to get out of the session. The majority indicated that they wanted to know what tests were available and what the risks of these tests were. Nearly half of them said they wanted reassurance about something. Few responses contained specific points on which clarification was wanted. For example, they asked about risks of tests, but did not specifically ask about miscarriage risk, risks of damaging the fetus or risks of damaging the mother. Very few women mentioned the accuracy of the test, and they did not distinguish between false positives and false negatives. In short, the questions these women wanted answered were stated in a very general way and a less than conscientious counsellor might feel that she had done her job by naming the tests, giving their respective miscarriage risks and reassuring a woman that she could have a test.

So why don't women mention specifics when asked what they want to learn at the session? The answer may be for the same reason as most of us ask few specific questions about a car or house survey. One has to know a lot about a subject in order to know what to ask. It is the responsibility of the counsellor to answer all the questions that probably would be asked if the pregnant woman knew more about the technology. People are unlikely to ask about the rate of culture failure if they do not know that the sample is cultured or that cultures sometimes fail.

Only a tiny number of women said they would like to know what conditions the tests could or could not identify and what their risks were for these conditions. Perhaps they thought, as Sally did, that an amniocentesis or chorionic villus sampling could detect all abnormalities. Sally said '...I want to be sure that the baby that I have is completely healthy and normal, otherwise I am not keeping it...'. It is the job of the counsellor to ensure that the woman does not leave the counselling session with this misapprehension as Caroline did. Caroline had an amniocentesis for advanced maternal age. The results were normal, but after she received the results an anomaly scan showed that her baby had cystic lungs and that the prognosis was very poor. She was extremely angry and repeatedly said that this could not be so, as the amniocentesis result was normal.

It is not always easy to convince women that normal amniocentesis results only rule out specified abnormalities. As many women said, they came to get reassurance and they may not easily take on board the fact that the reassurance is only partial. However, this problem is greatly compounded if the counsellor is loath to mention the limitations of the test. Collusion can occur between counsellor and counsellee. More than one woman has been told that the tests are 'just to make sure your baby is normal'.

CASE STUDIES

It may seem negative to dwell on all the times when counselling is not entirely satisfactory instead of applauding ourselves for all the very good counselling which takes place. However, none of us is perfect; we could all improve, and it is a fact that looking at our own and other people's shortcomings is often a way of working towards that improvement. With this in mind, the reader is invited to consider the following cases gathered over many years from many sources.

Case study 1

Rebecca was a Jehovah's Witness expecting her first child. She refused the offer of an alpha fetoprotein test because she said that she would not contemplate terminating a pregnancy for any reason and therefore did not wish to know if there was a fetal abnormality. She did, however, have an ultrasound scan at about 18 weeks of pregnancy, when anencephaly was diagnosed. Like most women, she did not have counselling prior to the scan and was unaware that one of the main reasons for the scan was to look for fetal anomalies. She and her partner felt very angry about the diagnosis having been made. Her right not to know had not been honoured. She had not been given the necessary information with which to decide whether or not to have a scan. She carried her baby to term in what was naturally a terribly stressful pregnancy.

Case study 2

Sandra was 35 years old. She had two healthy daughters and had suffered one late miscarriage. She was very pleased to find herself pregnant with a third child but feared that her luck might have run out and that this child might suffer from Down syndrome. She asked for an amniocentesis but was counselled that she was too young because at her age the test was more likely to cause a miscarriage than it was to detect a Down syndrome fetus. She pointed out that she knew how traumatic a late miscarriage could be but that she felt this did not begin to compare with the trauma of having a Down syndrome child and therefore she still wanted the test. The counsellor made the decision for her, refusing the amniocentesis. She worried for the entire pregnancy, but fortunately gave birth to a healthy son.

Case study 3

Beverly was a 39-year-old woman who had been trying unsuccessfully for many years to become pregnant. She finally became pregnant as a result of *in vitro* fertilization. At 16 weeks she had an amniocentesis which revealed that her fetus had Down syndrome. Beverly and her partner requested genetic counselling so that they could find out more about Down syndrome. After hearing what the geneticist had to say, they said that it wasn't so bad and that they had thought the amniocentesis was being done to test for serious abnormalities. They said that they would rather have a Down syndrome baby than no baby, and they decided to carry on with the pregnancy. It appeared that although the pregnancy had been very hard to achieve, Beverly had received only cursory pre-test counselling. It is questionable whether she would have decided to have an amniocentesis with the attendant risk of pregnancy loss if she had fully understood the purpose of it.

Case study 4

Perhaps the saddest case of all is Evelyn. Evelyn was a 24-year-old woman with two healthy children. In her third

pregnancy she had serum alpha fetoprotein screening for spina
bifida and was told that she was not at increased risk for
spina bifida. Some weeks later she was told that because her
serum alpha fetoprotein was low, she was at increased risk for
Down syndrome. The risk was not very high but was about
four times higher than her age risk alone. She was offered an
amniocentesis but became so upset about the possibility of
Down syndrome that she had the pregnancy terminated. Later
she became very distressed when she realized that in all likelihood she had aborted a normal baby. She claimed that she
had not been aware that the alpha fetoprotein test could provide any information about the chances of the baby having
Down syndrome and that this contributed to her sense of
shock and anxiety when she was suddenly told that she had
a raised risk for Down syndrome. It would appear either that
she was not given the relevant information about the screening
test or that she did not take in the information. In either case,
counselling before screening had been ineffective.

These cases are examples of counselling gone wrong at many
different levels. Perhaps one of the main problems that they all
had in common was that the counsellor was not really listening
to what the woman said or was not responding to non-verbal
cues.

For example, Rebecca said that she did not want to know if
the baby had an abnormality. She may have said that in reply to
an invitation to have an alpha fetoprotein test, but it remained
equally true for other tests. If the purpose of the scan had been
explained to her, she might have opted to have it, but she might
instead have decided against it. If she had decided to have the
scan and then received unwanted information, she might at least
have felt less as if she had been assaulted.

Sandra felt that the counsellor was deaf to all that she said,
because the reply always came back in the same simple formula
– 'the test is more likely to cause a miscarriage than it is to detect
Down syndrome' – as if the counsellor had not heard what she
had said about the relative meaning of the two events to her. If
the test was to be refused, the counsellor might have at least
acknowledged her anxiety.

Beverly must have made it obvious during the course of her

in vitro fertilization treatment how desperate she was to have a child, obvious that is to someone who was able to listen and to pick up cues. She certainly would have made it clear if a counsellor had explained the purpose of amniocentesis to her and had asked her how she felt about taking a risk with the pregnancy.

It is very likely that Evelyn gave some indication (verbal or non-verbal) of her extreme anxiety when she was offered the amniocentesis because of her low alpha fetoprotein result. Perhaps if this anxiety had been acknowledged and she had been encouraged to talk about it, she would have decided to carry on with the pregnancy. On the other hand, perhaps she was somehow looking for an excuse to terminate it and latched on to that one. In that case, it would have been better if she could have been gently led to explore why she really wanted to end the pregnancy.

THE IMPORTANCE OF LISTENING

Listening is a skill that some people seem to have in abundance and other people seem to lack in equal abundance! To some extent the skill or lack of it may be due to the individual's personality, life experiences and so on. However, it is also a skill which can be learned. It is an unfortunate fact, however, that many health workers finish their training without acquiring the ability to really listen and it is this inability which so often causes problems in the counselling situation.

CONCLUSION

We have seen that in pre-test counselling, as in all areas of life, there is a gap between how things are and how we would like them to be. This is not a cause for despair, but it is a cause for every one of us who is involved in this area to evaluate our own work and to think how we can improve it. For each of us the answer will be slightly different. For some it might be a short course to improve listening skills, for others it might be becoming better informed about the tests available. Most of us could improve upon the written literature which is given to women and could look into acquiring literature in other relevant languages. In the end, the most important thing we can do is to keep in mind that the people are important, and that the technology is there to serve the people rather than the other way around.

REFERENCES

Abramsky, L. and Rodeck, C.H. (1991) Women's choices for fetal chromosome analysis. *Prenatal Diagnosis*, **11**, 23–28.

Canadian Collaborative CVS-Amniocentesis Clinical Trial Group (1989) Multicentre randomized clinical trial of chorionic villus sampling and amniocentesis. *Lancet*, **i**, 1–6.

Chitty, L.S., Hunt, G.H., Moore, J. and Lobb, M.O. (1991) Effectiveness of routine ultrasonography in detecting fetal structural abnormalities in a low risk population. *British Medical Journal*, **303**, 1165–1169.

Clarke, A. (1991) Is non-directive genetic counselling possible? *Lancet*, **338**, 998–1001.

Crawfurd, M. ((1983) Ethical and legal aspects of early prenatal diagnosis. *British Medical Bulletin*, **39**(4), 310–314.

Ferguson-Smith, M.A. (1983) Prenatal chromosome analysis and its impact on the birth incidence of chromosome disorders. *British Medical Bulletin*, **39**(4), 355–364.

Green, J.M. (1990) Calming or harming: a critical review of psychological effects of fetal diagnosis on pregnant women. *Galton Institute Occasional Papers*, Second series, No 2.

Harper, P.S. (1981) *Practical Genetic Counselling*, John Wright, Bristol.

Levi, S., Hyjazi, Y., Schaaps, J.P. *et al.* (1991) Sensitivity and specificity of routine antenatal screening for congenital anomalies by ultrasouond: the Belgian Multicentric Study. *Ultrasound in Obstetrics and Gynaecology*, **1**, 102–110.

Lippman-Hand, J.A. and Fraser, F.C. (1979) Genetic counselling – the post counselling period: Parents' perceptions of uncertainty. *American Journal of Medical Genetics*, **4**, 51–71.

Marteau, T.M., Slack, D.M.H., Kidd, J. and Shaw, R.W. (1992) Presenting a routine screening test in antenatal care: practice observed. *Public Health*, **106**, 131–141.

MRC Working Party on the Evaluation of Chorion Villus Sampling (1991) Medical Research Council European trial of chorion villus sampling. *Lancet*, **337**, 1491–1499.

Rodeck, C.H. and Nicolaides, K.H. (1983), Fetoscopy and fetal tissue sampling. *British Medical Bulletin*, **39**(4), 332–337.

Rothman, B.K. (1986) *The Tentative Pregnancy: Prenatal Diagnosis and the Future of Motherhood*, Viking Penguin, New York.

Shirley, I.M., Bottomley, F. and Robinson, V.P. (1992) Routine radiographer screening for fetal abnormalities by ultrasound in an unselected low risk population. *British Journal of Radiology*, **65**(775), 564–569.

Sjogren, B. and Uddenberg, N. (1988) Decision making during the prenatal diagnostic procedure. A questionnaire and interview study of 211 women participating in prenatal diagnosis. *Prenatal Diagnosis*, **8**, 263–273.

Turnbull, A.C. and Mackenzie, I.Z. (1983) Second-trimester amnio-centesis and termination of pregnancy. *British Medical Bulletin*, **39(4)**, 315–321.

6

Difficult decisions in prenatal diagnosis

Christine Garrett and Lyn Carlton

Decisions in prenatal diagnosis are difficult when the diagnosis is clear. How much more difficult it is when there is only a risk of abnormality, or where the effects of the abnormality cannot be predicted. This chapter will explore some of these situations, the ways in which couples come to a decision and the role of the counsellor in helping them to decide.

UNSUSPECTED CHROMOSOME ABNORMALITIES

Prenatal diagnosis is usually performed because of concern about a particular chromosomal abnormality, most commonly Down syndrome, trisomy 21. Prenatal diagnosis counselling should include explanation of the possibility that other chromosome abnormalities may also be detected. Trisomy 18 or trisomy 13, both lethal abnormalities, are conditions where the outcome can be predicted and the choice facing the couple is usually clear. This is not so when a sex chromosome trisomy, an apparently balanced structural rearrangement or mosaicism is detected. In such cases the outcome may be difficult to predict and, while many such babies may be entirely normal, some may suffer from significant handicap. The counsellor needs to be aware of the effects of these chromosome abnormalities in order to give the couple the most reliable information on which to base their decision as to whether to continue the pregnancy. These problems are considered in more detail below.

Sex chromosome abnormalities

Klinefelter syndrome

Males with XXY chromosomes, Klinefelter syndrome, are found in approximately 1 in 1000 male births (Editorial, 1988). Not long ago the traditional textbook description of Klinefelter syndrome was of a mentally retarded male, lacking in male secondary sexual characteristics and with breast enlargement – an alarming prospect for future parents. This picture resulted from a bias in selection, since originally only those with the most severe manifestations were karyotyped, and the true extent of the effects of Klinefelter syndrome has only recently emerged from prospective studies involving long-term follow up of babies identified by newborn surveys (Ratcliffe, Butler and James, 1990; Robinson *et al.*, 1990; Leonard, 1990). Performance intelligence quotient scores are normal but there is a 10–20 point reduction in verbal skills, with significant problems in expressive language. While most boys attend normal schools, the speech and language disorder may require speech therapy. Men with Klinefelter syndrome are invariably infertile. Tall stature is a feature but there is no increase in congenital malformations. Gynaecomastia may occur, but rarely requires surgery. The chance of homosexuality or transsexualism is not increased, although diminished potency or libido may require treatment with testosterone replacement. There is a tendency towards passive behaviour characterized by lack of self esteem, shyness and emotional immaturity. However, preliminary data suggest that most affected males manage well with respect to social adjustment and socioeconomic status.

Triple X syndrome

In the Triple X syndrome the baby is female and has an extra X chromosome, an abnormality found in approximately 1 in 1000 female births. As with Klinefelter syndrome, early reports tended to exaggerate the effects of the extra X chromosome, because ascertainment was biased in favour of individuals who were karyotyped because of significant problems. Prospective studies on girls diagnosed by screening at birth give a more accurate picture (Ratcliffe, Butler and James, 1990; Leonard, 1990; Linden,

Bender and Harmon, 1988). There are no distinguishing features at birth but as they grow older affected individuals become relatively tall with long legs, with a slightly reduced head circumference. Sexual development is usually normal and many women with triple X syndrome are fertile. However there may be an increased incidence of infertility and premature menopause, and women with triple X syndrome are probably more likely to have chromosomally abnormal offspring, particularly with an extra X chromosome. The main cause for concern is the possible effects on the child's future intellectual development and personality. Delay in speech and language development are common, and speech therapy is often necessary. Lack of coordination, poor academic performance and immature behaviour may persist throughout childhood and overall intelligence quotient is reduced by around 10 points. Behavioural problems are common and few achieve academic success. The risk of psychotic disorders may be increased.

Extra Y chromosome

An extra Y chromosome, XYY, is found in approximately 1 in 1000 male births and is not associated with raised maternal or paternal age. This finding on amniocentesis may present the parents with a dilemma, not least because of the association in the older medical literature of this condition with criminality. Again, the true picture is beginning to emerge from data built up from long-term follow up of boys with XYY ascertained by newborn surveys (Ratcliffe, Butler and James, 1990; Leonard, 1990; Robinson *et al.*, 1990). Affected boys are physically indistinguishable from the general population, but tend to be taller than average. Behaviour problems are frequent in childhood, with temper tantrums and hyperactivity, and speech development may be delayed. Intelligence is 10–15 points less than that of their normal siblings and verbal intelligence quotient is affected more than performance. Many XYY men have fathered children who are chromosomally normal but there is probably an increased risk of a chromosomal abnormality, including XYY, in their offspring.

Turner syndrome

Absence of a sex chromosome, 45,X, causes Turner syndrome. The main features are short stature, infertility, and mild specific learning difficulties (Connor, 1986). The incidence is 1 in 10 000 newborn girls, but is much higher at conception, representing nearly 2% of conceptions. Over 99% abort spontaneously, most in the first trimester. It should be explained to the parents when a diagnosis of Turner syndrome is made at amniocentesis that less than a fifth will survive to term. For those diagnosed by chorionic villus sampling this figure is probably less than 1%. Congenital malformations are found more frequently in Turner syndrome, especially coarctation of the aorta and renal malformations. Mean adult height is 143 cm (4 ft 9 in), but treatment with low dose oestrogens and growth hormone may be beneficial in increasing final height (Dean, 1991). The ovaries are present in fetal life but then degenerate to streaks of tissue, resulting in amenorrhoea and lack of secondary sex characteristics. Occasionally a woman with Turner syndrome may menstruate, and rarely pregnancy may occur, although the offspring may be abnormal. Usually hormone replacement therapy is required in order to produce secondary sexual characteristics. Since the uterus is present, pregnancy is possible using ovum donation (Serhal and Craft, 1989). As in the other sex chromosome abnormalities, ascertainment bias originally led to an overestimate of the incidence of intellectual problems. The intelligence quotient is normal except that verbal ability tends to exceed performance, and visuospatial perceptual difficulties are common. Low self-esteem and depression may be a problem (Robinson *et al.*, 1990).

Outcome of pregnancies with a sex chromosome abnormality

When a sex chromosome abnormality is discovered prenatally, the parents should be offered expert counselling. This should include an explanation of the chromosome abnormality and information about the anticipated effects, based on the prospective studies following newborn surveys. Many parents ask to see relevant literature and photographs, but there is little suitable literature available at present and text books tend to show extreme examples which may give a biased view. Showing photographs of patients whose parents have given their permission presents a more realistic picture (Clayton-Smith, Andrews and Donnai, 1989). For parents facing a decision as to whether to continue the pregnancy, the main issues are the possibility of congenital abnormalities, the risk of mental retardation, the concern about behavioural problems and the prospects for establishing sexual identity, future sexual relationships and a successful family life. In discussions with parents, the future happiness of the child is a major consideration, as are the effects on the well-being of the parents and other siblings.

There is wide variation in reports of the outcome of pregnancies with prenatally diagnosed sex chromosome abnormalities. In a series from Denmark, 80% of such pregnancies were terminated (Nielsen *et al.*, 1986), from Finland, 88%, from the United Kingdom, 56%, and from a review of other reports, 62% (Holmes-Seidle, Ryyanen and Lindenbaum, 1987). Another series from the United Kingdom reports that 63% of pregnancies were terminated (Clayton-Smith, Andrews and Donnai, 1989). There is a tendency for more parents to opt to continue the pregnancy as more information from prospective studies becomes available (Holmes-Seidle, Ryyanen and Lindenbaum, 1987).

When confronted with a diagnosis of Turner syndrome prenatally the parents may opt to continue the pregnancy, especially when they have been given the full information (Connor, 1986). In one series, however, all pregnancies with an abnormal ultrasound were terminated. One-third of the remainder continued and all of these were mosaics with a normal cell line, who would be expected to show milder effect (Holmes-Seidle, Ryyanen and Lindenbaum, 1987). The observation that termination is more commonly chosen for Turner syndrome and for Klinefelter syndrome could indicate that the prospect of infertility in an offspring is of major concern (Evans, MacDonald and Hamilton 1990). Parents are more inclined to continue the pregnancy with triple X than with Klinefelter syndrome. This may be due to anxieties about future infertility in Klinefelter syndrome but may also be due to a perception in society, invalid as it may be, that intellectual achievement and socioeconomic success are more important for a boy than a girl. Where the fetus has an XYY karyotype, decisions as to whether to continue the pregnancy are determined largely by the parents' expectations for their child and their concern that he might be disadvantaged in life (particularly important for a boy, they may feel) and that psychological difficulties may cause him unhappiness.

Parents are concerned as to when the child should be told about the abnormality, and who else might be told. This may lead to discussion as to whether problems are more likely to occur if they are expected – the self-fulfilling prophesy (Puck, 1981). To balance this, there is the view that early intervention to provide help for speech or behavioural problems, while requiring the support of teachers and others outside the family, may nevertheless be beneficial. There is some evidence that the outcome is better where the abnormality is diagnosed prenatally (Robinson, Bender and Linden, 1992). This may be due in part to the supportive family environment and 'positive parenting' of these children, where the parents have made a conscious decision to continue.

Structural rearrangements

Chromosomes are prone to breakage and rejoining, which may give rise to a structural rearrangement, usually a translocation or inversion. Such rearrangements are found in about 1 in 1600 amniocenteses and are the cause of considerable anxiety. If the rearrangement appears to be balanced, meaning that no active genetic material has been lost or added, and is found in one of the parents, there should be no harmful effects. However, if it has occurred *de novo* – out of the blue – and is not found in either parent it could cause congenital abnormalities or mental retardation. This is because the rearrangement may not really be balanced, a small segment of chromosome having been gained or lost, or the break may have occurred within or close to a gene, causing disruption of its function. The phenotypic effects are unpredictable and this leads to great difficulty for the parents in assessing whether or not to terminate the pregnancy.

Apparently balanced chromosome rearrangements may be associated with mental retardation and congenital malformations (Jacobs, 1974). The risk of abnormality is difficult to estimate because of ascertainment bias (Donnai, 1989) and can only be reliably assessed by follow-up of *de novo* translocations detected by chance prenatally. The incidence of congenital abnormalities and mental retardation in one follow-up series was found to be increased two to three times over the general population risk

(Warburton, 1991). This is lower than previous studies which have suggested a risk of up to 10% (Hsu, 1986). Problems common to all these studies have been the small numbers of cases, the short length of follow-up, and the difficulty in assessing the presence of an abnormality if the pregnancy was terminated. There is still a need for further information on which to base figures for counselling, and this is the subject of an ongoing study (Donnai, 1989).

In one survey, about 25% of couples elected to terminate the pregnancy following counselling (Warburton, 1991). In another small series from a centre giving an optimistic prognosis only one out of eight pregnancies was terminated, and this was for an abnormality detected on ultrasound. Some reassurance can be offered if high resolution ultrasound examination is normal as this would be expected to detect one-third of abnormalities (Warburton, 1991).

Supernumary marker chromosomes

A supernumary marker chromosome (an extra chromosome fragment) discovered prenatally causes similar difficulties to a structural rearrangement. Urgent karyotyping of the parents is needed and if one of the parents has the same supernumary marker it is presumed to be genetically inactive, with no increased risk of fetal abnormality. *De novo* markers are found in around 1 in 2500 amniocenteses and are associated with congenital malformations and mental handicap, but this risk is difficult to assess because of ascertainment bias. Prospective studies of *de novo* markers found at amniocentesis showed an overall risk of abnormality of 13% (Warburton, 1991). Special cytogenetic techniques to identify the chromosome are becoming available which may allow for more accurate risk estimation to be given in future (Verschraegen-Spae *et al.*, 1993). Almost half of the pregnancies where a *de novo* marker was identified prenatally were terminated, reflecting the perception of the counsellors that the risk of abnormality is high (Warburton, 1991).

Mosaicism

Chromosome mosaicism is the mixture of two or more cell lines with different chromosome constitutions. Mosaicism found prenatally can cause difficulties in interpretation in the laboratory and causes anxiety in parents and counsellors. The problem is whether the abnormal cells are present in the fetus and, if so, how this might affect the baby. The possibility of finding mosaicism should be explained during prenatal diagnosis counselling. True mosaicism occurs in about 1 in 500 amniocenteses (Hsu *et al.*, 1992), and even more frequently in chorionic villus sampling material since mosaicism is more common in the placenta than in the fetus. This confined chorionic mosaicism may arise early in embryonic development, or could arise from a vanishing twin (Gardner and Sutherland, 1989).

Specific details about the degree and type of mosaicism will influence the counselling given to the patient and the extent to which further investigation is performed. The presence of an abnormality on high resolution ultrasound is likely to influence any decision regarding termination. Amniocentesis to confirm mosaicism found at chorionic villus sampling may be useful, but repeat amniocentesis is usually not helpful since a normal result does not invalidate the findings of the previous test. Fetal blood sampling may yield further information but is associated with a small risk of miscarriage and does not exclude mosaicism completely, even if all the cells sampled are normal (Gosden, Nicolaides and Rodeck, 1988). In one series, termination was performed in 40% of cases of true mosaicism and was more likely in autosomal than sex chromosome mosaicism (Hsu *et al.*, 1992).

THE FETUS AT RISK OF BEING AFFECTED

There are several circumstances where the fetus is at risk of having a handicap but is not definitely known to be affected. Parents may find it very difficult to decide whether the risk is sufficiently serious to warrant termination of the pregnancy, and may find counselling helpful.

This situation may arise if the mother is exposed to a possible teratogen early in the pregnancy. Parents need to know what defects might occur and the likelihood of the baby being affected. Some couples feel that any increased risk of abnormality is unacceptable and will opt for termination, whereas others wish to continue unless they are told that the baby is definitely abnormal.

Many couples who are at risk of having a son with Duchenne

muscular dystrophy can now be offered accurate prenatal diagnosis, either by direct detection of the mutation or by linkage
analysis. There are still couples for whom this is not possible
and the only form of prenatal diagnosis is fetal sexing, with the
option of termination if the fetus is male. A mother who has
grown up with affected brothers may feel very strongly that she
does not wish to take any risk, and may be prepared to go
through more than one termination rather than have to face
having an affected son herself. The options are similar if the
mother is at risk of being a carrier for an X-linked condition for
which there is no accurate prenatal diagnosis as yet, for example
some forms of X-linked mental retardation.

Another situation where couples may opt for termination
because of a risk that the baby could have inherited a genetic
disorder occurs if one of the couple has a parent with Huntington's disease and does not wish to risk passing on the condition
to the child. Prenatal diagnosis of Huntington's disease has been
possible for several years in informative families using linkage
analysis, and can now be achieved by direct detection of the
mutation in the gene. Where the couple do not wish to undergo
predictive testing themselves, prenatal exclusion of the gene may
be offered. If the fetus is shown to have inherited a chromosome
from the affected grandparent, the baby will have a high risk,
approaching 50%, of having the Huntington gene and the couple
may opt for termination (Tyler *et al.*, 1990). This is acceptable to
couples who feel that they could not risk passing on the condition, but nevertheless have a strong desire for a child. They
may be prepared to go through more than one termination to
achieve this.

FACTORS AFFECTING DECISIONS REGARDING TERMINATION
OF PREGNANCY WHERE THE DIAGNOSIS OR PROGNOSIS IS
UNCERTAIN

All parents faced with the choice of whether or not to terminate
a pregnancy for fetal abnormality have to make a very difficult
decision. Not all will chose termination, even where prenatal
diagnosis was done in order to detect the abnormality found
(Verp *et al.*, 1988). Many factors influence the parents' decision.
When the diagnosis or prognosis is unclear, as in the situations

described above, the decision may cause great anguish. The counsellor has to provide a full and accurate explanation of the problem, as well as helping in the decision-making process and supporting the parents afterwards. A number of studies have tried to identify factors influencing the decision. While these are able to identify trends, it must be remembered that for each pregnancy the circumstances are unique and the outcome will depend not only on the abnormality in the baby, but also on the significance of the pregnancy to that particular couple, who have invested their future aspirations in their coming child.

The severity of the problem

One of the main factors in the parents' decision was the severity of the abnormality. When the prognosis was severe, such as for autosomal trisomy, 93% of pregnancies were terminated, whereas in questionable abnormalities, such as apparently balanced trans-locations, 27% of parents opted for termination (Drugan *et al.*, 1990). As discussed previously, the presence of a congenital abnormality and the prospect of future infertility may influence the decision as to whether to terminate the pregnancy for a sex chromosome abnormality. The pregnancy is more likely to continue where mosaicism is present, since the effects would be expected to be milder (Robinson *et al.*, 1990; Holmes-Seidle, Ryyanen and Lindenbaum, 1987).

Experience of the condition

The couple's previous knowledge or experience of the condition may affect their decision. It is probably easier if they have experience of the problem in their own family or acquaintance as they will be aware of the burdens involved. This is apparent where a woman who has had a brother with Duchenne muscular dystrophy may prefer to terminate all pregnancies with a male fetus, rather than risk having an affected child. In other, more variable, conditions their view will be coloured by the severity in the person they have known, which might not be typical. Because of this variation, it may not always be helpful for a couple contemplating termination for an abnormality to make contact with affected families.

Gestational age

A decision to terminate the pregnancy after diagnosis of a chromosomal abnormality by chorionic villus sampling in the first trimester, when there is less emotional involvement with the fetus, would be expected to be less difficult than following amniocentesis. There is some evidence for this from one series, where 98% of affected pregnancies diagnosed by chorionic villus sampling were terminated, whereas 78% diagnosed by amniocentesis were terminated (Verp *et al.*, 1988). Another survey found no difference, although this could be biased, as the two methods were not randomly assigned (Drugan *et al.*, 1990). Termination might be less difficult in the first trimester, when there is more privacy and less pressure from family and friends. The procedure is safer and less frightening and might be expected to lead to less emotional sequelae. This is not necessarily the case, and the baby may be imagined as a real person from very early in pregnancy. Early termination may deny the possibility of seeing and holding the baby, and this may make the loss harder to bear (Seller *et al.*, 1993).

The effect of ultrasound

The presence of structural abnormality on ultrasound, having a more direct impact than an abnormal karyotype, is a highly significant factor in the decision to opt for termination (Holmes-Seidle *et al.*, 1987; Drugan *et al.*, 1990). On the other hand, since ultrasound enhances early parental bonding, a normal ultrasound scan reinforces the decision to continue the pregnancy when the risk of abnormality is low. Couples undergoing prenatal diagnosis who know beforehand that they may terminate the pregnancy (for example, for Duchenne muscular dystrophy) may wish to avoid seeing the baby on the scan, so that the decision to terminate the pregnancy is not made even more difficult.

Family structure

Older parents are less likely to terminate the pregnancy for a sex chromosome abnormality, possibly because they have less chance of having another baby and more chance of having one with a severe abnormality next time (Holmes-Seidle *et al.*, 1987). Parents continuing the pregnancy had more children than those choosing termination. This could be related to their age, or perhaps it reflects a greater desire for children in some parents. Alternatively, they may not have such high expectations of their offspring if these are already fulfilled by their previous children.

Socioeconomic and cultural factors

Socioeconomic and cultural factors inevitably affect the parents' decision . The more affluent parents in one series from the United States were more likely to terminate the pregnancy with a sex chromosome abnormality (Tannenbaum *et al.*, 1986). The financial circumstances of the family may be influential. One mother felt unable to continue the pregnancy when the baby was found to have Klinefelter syndrome. She was concerned that the demands of a child with behaviour problems or special needs would conflict with her job, and as a single parent she would risk losing her only means of economic support.

Psychological factors

There are many other factors regarding the couple's feelings about the pregnancy which might be expected to influence their decision. The pregnancy may have been unplanned and unwelcome, and paradoxically this may add to feelings of guilt if an abnormality is found, with greater reluctance to terminate the pregnancy. This may also occur if there is revival of guilt feelings regarding a previous termination for social reasons. The pregnancy may be particularly precious, having been achieved after years of infertility, or after the loss of a previous pregnancy or child, or courageously in the face of a high risk of abnormality, or as a last chance in older parents. The baby's sex may be influential if it fulfils the desire for a boy or girl.

The couple may have strong religious or moral objections to termination, or feel revulsion towards it, or believe that it prevents nature taking its course. There is fear of the physical and long-term emotional burdens of termination, and fear of others knowing and being censorious.

These factors have to be weighed against the fear of having a handicapped child, and the desire to prevent it from suffering, and concern about the effect on' other siblings and the relationships within the family. Couples question their ability to cope, physically, emotionally and financially, with the extra burdens. They may have very high expectations for their child's future, particularly for a first child, which a handicapped child could not fulfil. This may have influenced the decision of one older childless couple to terminate the pregnancy when the baby was found to have an XYY karyotype. Yet another mother with fewer socioeconomic advantages and several children, one of whom had learning difficulties, decided to continue as she knew she would be able to cope.

Some parents tend to polarize their perceptions of the problem with the baby. Those who feel either that any increased risk of abnormality is unacceptable, or that they would not wish to terminate the pregnancy without knowing that the baby would be severely affected, seem to find it easier to come to a decision.

The attitudes of others

Couples may be influenced by the attitudes of others. A woman's decision to terminate the pregnancy will depend on her partner's feelings, which she may feel have equal weight to her own. Some partners may have strong views against termination which may sway her decision. Others feel that it is for her to decide as she is more closely involved, and support her in her decision. Couples want to know how their decision will be viewed objectively by others, and often ask what the counsellor would do, or what most other couples have done in their situation. The counsellor should try to be non-directive, but information about what others have decided may help the couple to test the validity of their decision. There may be a danger here of seeming to exert social pressures on the couple.

The effect of counselling

The decision to terminate is also influenced by the counselling received. Parents are more likely to continue the pregnancy when counselled by a geneticist rather than an obstetrician (Holmes-Seidle, Ryyanen and Lindenbaum, 1987). Geneticists would be expected to be better informed as to the prognosis in sex chromosome abnormality and can offer more encouraging information from prospective studies. They may be more inclined to offer non-directive counselling, with the aim of preserving the parents' autonomy.

The task of advising a couple faced with an unexpected abnormality of uncertain significance in pregnancy is one of the most difficult in genetic counselling. The counsellor should try to see the couple together, without delay, and should try to reduce their level of stress. The information to be communicated is often complex and the lack of certainty is frustrating to both the parents and counsellor. There is often little time for reflection, but the counsellor should try to provide the framework for the couple to make their decision and support them afterwards. The role of the counsellor and the decision-making process itself are explored more fully below.

THE ROLE OF THE COUNSELLOR IN DECISION MAKING

Counselling can be simply defined as the process by which one person helps another to resolve a difficulty and decide on an appropriate course of action. The Oxford Dictionary includes the phrases 'give advice' and 'recommend' within its definition. The emphasis in most counselling situations now is towards a non-directive approach, which facilitates the process while allowing the client the space and freedom to make his/her own decisions. How far this can apply in prenatal diagnosis is debatable (Clarke, 1991; Pembrey, 1991). A number of models exist that define the stages in counselling, some more complex than others. This useful and simple version reduces the process to three stages (Egan, 1986).

- Identify and clarify the problem situations.
- Set the goals – develop and choose the preferred scenarios.
- Action – move towards preferred scenarios.

Within this basic framework a wide range of different approaches might be employed, but the aim should always be to assist the client to make a valid and autonomous decision. As an aid to determining whether this has been achieved, the Hastings Centre in the United States proposed the following short checklist of considerations that the client needs to be aware of and understand (Miller, 1981).

- There is no such thing as 'free action'. There will always be pressures from somewhere and these need to be recognized.
- There must be a period of effective deliberation.
- The authenticity of any decision must be checked by the client so that he/she is not acting out of character or contrary to his/her own needs.
- There needs to be moral reflection in which the client decides whether the action proposed is reasonable, informed, right for him/her, and something he/she can live with.

Communicating risk figures

Genetic counselling deals with people who are in search of some certainty. There is none, and the most that can be offered is possible outcomes and their probable occurrence. The counsellor has to appreciate that the language of figures is as fraught with ambiguity as any other. To further confuse matters, there is a lack of consensus among practitioners regarding the level of probability conveyed by the descriptive words such as 'high', 'moderate' and 'low' (Parsons and Atkinson 1992). The strategies used in comprehending risk figures have an impact on what the figures mean. One person looks at a risk of 10% of 1 000 000 people as a large number of people and therefore a high risk, another as analogous to 10% off in a sale – a small saving, therefore a low risk (Kessler and Levine, 1987). Furthermore, there is no guarantee that the client will be able to understand the meaning of the figures at all, and may believe that a 1 in 20 risk of abnormality is preferable to 1 in 200. The severity of a disorder can affect the perception of the actual risk figure, and a low risk of severe disorder may actually be seen as a high risk (Frets *et al.*, 1990). The whole validity of risk measurement is questionable, when the actual figure may be of less concern to the patient than the fact that they are in a state of being at risk (Lippman-Hand and Fraser, 1979). Awareness of these problems will help the counsellor to clarify the decision facing the patient.

Models for decision making

Having to address a complex problem can be psychologically paralysing. It is common for people to postpone the decision for as long as possible. A decision taken at the last moment will often be impulsive, failing to take account of all the relevant factors. Couples need time to make decisions about termination of pregnancy, but they also need an end point so that a decision to continue is not made by default – in effect having made no decision.

The more complex the problem, the more difficult it is to resolve. Firstly, short-term memory is stretched by having to keep track of several different alternatives, and people will often forget one aspect while dealing with others. Secondly, direct comparison between alternative options can be problematic when the outcomes are dissimilar in kind. Parents facing termination may have to weigh the consequences of losing a healthy baby against the long-term stress of having an affected child. The literature on decision making contains a number of sophisticated tools intended to aid the decision-making process, some of which have been applied to genetic counselling.

A model resembling Egan's three-stage counselling model requires strict, sequential working through in order to reach a 'high quality' decision, with recognition of the effect of stress on the client's ability to make a decision (Janis and Mann, 1977). Another model requires that recognition of the five sequential stages of the coping response (shock and denial, anxiety, anger and guilt, depression and psychological homoeostasis) are necessary before a valid decision can be made (Falek, 1984).

A less structured approach favours the use of 'worst case scenarios' as a test of the client's ability to cope, emphasizing the tendency for clients to process the complex issues of risk into a binary form and adopt a broad view of the consequences of having an affected child (Lipmann-Hand and Fraser, 1979).

A common technique uses a value or utility for each possible outcome. Utilities are calculated by multiplying the probability of the outcome by a numeric measure of the desirability of that outcome for the client. In complex situations a 'decision tree' can be drawn up which shows the various possible consequences of the options open to the client, each carrying its own utility. The course of action which results in the highest utility is the one, rationally and logically speaking, which the client should follow (Zarin and Pauker, 1984). An obvious benefit of this approach is that the client only needs to consider one set of circumstances at a time, thus overcoming the limits of memory. However, the technique fails because of the difficulties in ascribing meaningful numeric values to outcomes, especially when many of these involve considerations that are uncertain and intangible.

Several models in the literature get away from the quantitative analysis of the decision tree. In one approach (Vleck, 1987), desirability is weighed against expected stress. A situation is analysed in terms of desirable and undesirable outcomes and the practical and emotional demands and coping abilities associated with them. The client determines the acceptability of various possible scenarios, including the best scenario, which helps to put into perspective other alternatives. For instance, parents need to be aware of the expectations they may have for their offspring in order to assess how they would cope should the disorder make these impossible to fulfil.

Increasingly, there is recognition that decision-aiding processes need to take account of the various medical, psychological, social, religious, familial and financial implications of the decision. Human behaviour is not always a 'goal-oriented intellectual process' but rather a simpler or more direct procedure of permitting immediate rewards and punishments to dictate direction (Cross and Guyer, 1980). A client at risk of transmitting Huntington disease who once felt that prenatal exclusion testing was a moral obligation on anyone in her position changed her mind because of the strain it might put on her new relationship. In this case, the immediate rewards of a stress-free relationship overrode the ethical certainties and the threat of future punishment.

Psychological and social factors

A different approach is the idea of an 'interpretive perspective' (Parsons, 1993). This starts from the acceptance of the beliefs and 'prior biography' the client brings to the counselling situation. Parsons points out that the client is not an empty container waiting to be filled with information. Her approach respects the ability of the client to 'negotiate and construct' his/her life around the consequences of genetic disease. It does not assume the prime importance of risks, and is open to recognizing the many factors which influence the client.

Although much of the work in this field remains inconclusive and sometimes contradictory, a broad consensus is beginning to emerge. It is evident that research in relation to reproductive decision making is demonstrating a wide acceptance for a more holistic and client-centred approach. The prime need is to be flexible and to borrow any method that seems appropriate in a given situation. To work effectively, an underlying structure is needed. The Hastings checklist is succinct and comprehensive. It meets the same procedural objectives of other, more complex models, but by emphasizing the importance of authenticity and moral reflection, it ensures that the final decision is right for each individual client. Parsons's approach leads us to see the client as a person who brings to the counselling situation a past history and set of beliefs which are relevant to the decision they must make. The role of the counsellor then becomes that of a reliable informer and facilitator who works within the agenda that is set by the pre-existing plans and definitions that the family hold.

REFERENCES

Clarke, A. (1991) Is non-directive genetic counselling possible? *Lancet*, ii, 998–1001.

Clayton-Smith, J., Andrews, T. and Donnai, D. (1989) Genetic counselling and parental decisions following antenatal diagnosis of sex chromosome aneuploidies. *Journal of Obstetrics and Gynaecology*, 10, 5–7.

Connor, J.M.(1986) Prenatal diagnosis of the Turner syndrome; what to tell the parents. *British Medical Journal*, 293, 711–712.

Cross, J. and Guyer, M. (1980) *Social Traps*, University of Michigan Press, Ann Arbor, MI.

Dean, H. (1991) Growth hormone therapy in girls with Turner syndrome, in *Children and Young Adults with Sex Chromosome Aneuploidy*, (eds J.A. Evans, J.L. Hammerton and A. Robinson), Wiley-Liss for the National Foundation–March of Dimes, New York, pp. 239–234.

Donnai D. (1989) The clinical significance of *de novo* structural rearrangements and markers detected prenatally by amniocentesis. *Journal of Medical Genetics*, 26, 545.

Drugan, A., Greb, A., Johnson, M.P. *et al.* (1990) Determinants of parental decisions to abort for chromosome abnormalities. *Prenatal Diagnosis*, 10, 483–490.

Editorial (1988) Klinefelter's syndrome. *Lancet*, ii, 1316–1317.

Egan, G. (1986) *The Skilled Helper*, Brooks/Cole, California

Evans, J.A., MacDonald, K. and Hammerton, J.L. (1990) Sex chromosome anomalies: prenatal diagnosis and the need for continued prospective studies, in *Children and Young Adults with Sex Chromosome Aneuploidy*, (eds J.A. Evans, J.L. Hammerton and A. Robinson), Wiley-Liss for the National Foundation–March of Dimes, New York, pp. 273–281.

Falek, A. (1984) Sequential aspects of coping and other issues in decision making in genetic counselling, in *Psychological Aspects of Genetic*

Counselling, (eds A.E.H. Emery and I.M. Pullen), Academic Press, London, pp. 23–36.

Frets, P.G., Duivenvoorden, H.J., Verhage, F. *et al.* (1990) Factors influencing the reproductive decision after genetic counselling. *American Journal of Medical Genetics*, **35**, 496–502.

Gardner, R.J.M. and Sutherland, G.R. (1989) *Chromosome Abnormalities and Genetic Counselling*, Oxford Monographs on Medical Genetics 17, Oxford University Press, Oxford, p. 193.

Gosden, C.M., Nicolaides, K.H. and Rodeck, C.H. (1988) Fetal blood sampling in investigation of chromosome mosaicism in amniotic fluid cell culture. *Lancet*, **i**, 613–617.

Holmes-Seidle, M., Ryyanen, M. and Lindenbaum, R.H. (1987) Parental decisions regarding termination of pregnancy following prenatal detection of sex chromosome abnormality. *Prenatal Diagnosis*, **7**, 239–244.

Hsu, L.Y.F. (1986) Prenatal diagnosis of chromosome abnormalities, in *Genetic Disorders and the Fetus*, (ed. A. Milunsky), 2nd edn, Plenum Press, New York.

Hsu, L.Y.F., Kaffe, S., Jenkins, E.C. *et al.* (1992) Proposed guidelines for diagnosis of chromosome mosaicism in amniocytes based on data derived from chromosome mosaicism and pseudomosaicism studies. *Prenatal Diagnosis*, **12**, 555–573.

Jacobs, P. (1974) Correlation between euploid structural rearrangements and mental subnormality in humans. *Nature*, **249**, 164–165.

Janis, J. and Mann, L. (1977) *Decision Making: a Psychological Analysis of Conflict, Choice and Commitment*, Free Press, New York.

Kessler, S. and Levine, E.K. (1987) Psychological aspects of genetic counselling 4. The subjective assessment of probability. *American Journal of Medical Genetics*, **28**, 361–370.

Leonard, M.F. (1990) A prospective study of development of children with sex chromosome abnormalities, in *Children and Young Adults with Sex Chromosome Aneuploidy*, (eds J.A. Evans, J.L. Hammerton and A. Robinson), Wiley-Liss for the National Foundation–March of Dimes, New York, pp. 117–130.

Linden, M.G., Bender, B.G. and Harmon, R.J. (1988) 47,XXX: what is the prognosis? *Pediatrics*, **82**(4), 619–630.

Lippman-Hand, A. and Fraser, F.C. (1979) Genetic counselling – the post counselling period: 1. Parents' perceptions of uncertainty. *American Journal of Medical Genetics*, **4**, 51–71.

Miller, B.L. (1981) *Hastings Centre Report*, **11**(4), 22–28.

Nielsen, J., Wohlert, M., Faaborg-Andersen, J. *et al.* (1986) Chromosome examination of 20,222 newborn children: results from a 7.5 year study in Arhus, Denmark, in *Prospective Studies in Children with Sex Chromosome Aneuploidy*, (eds S.G. Ratcliffe and N. Paul),Wiley-Liss for the National Foundation–March of Dimes, New York, pp. 209–219.

Parsons, E.P. (1993) Genetic risk and reproduction. *Sociological Review*, **41**(4).

Parsons, E.P. and Atkinson, P.A. (1992) Lay construction of genetic risk. *Sociology of Health and Illness*, **14**(4), 437–455.

Pembrey, M. (1991) Non-directive genetic counselling. *Lancet*, **ii**, 1266–1267.

Puck, M.H. (1981) Some considerations bearing on the doctrine of self-fulfilling prophesy in sex chromosome aneuploidy. *American Journal of Medical Genetics*, **9**, 129–137.

Ratcliffe, S.G., Butler, G.E. and James, M. (1990) Edinburgh study of growth and development of children with sex chromosome abnormalities: IV, in *Children and Young Adults with Sex Chromosome Aneuploidy*, (eds J.A. Evans, J.L. Hammerton and A. Robinson), Wiley-Liss for the National Foundation–March of Dimes, New York, pp. 1–44.

Robinson, A., Bender, B.G., Linden, M.G. *et al.* (1990) Sex chromosome aneuploidy: the Denver prospective study, in *Children and Young Adults with Sex Chromosome Aneuploidy*, (eds J.A. Evans, J.L. Hammerton and A. Robinson), Wiley-Liss for the National Foundation–March of Dimes, New York, pp. 59–115.

Robinson, A., Bender, B.G. and Linden, M.G. (1992) Prognosis of prenatally diagnosed children with sex chromosome aneuploidy. *American Journal of Medical Genetics*, **44**, 365–368.

Seller, M., Barnes, C., Ross, S. *et al.* (1993) Grief and mid-trimester fetal loss. *Prenatal Diagnosis*, **13**, 341–348.

Serhal, P.F. and Craft, I.L. (1989) Oocyte donation in 60 patients. *Lancet*, **i**, 1185–1187.

Tannenbaum, H.L., Perlis, T.E., Arbeitel, B.E. and Hsu, L.Y.F. (1986) Analysis of decision to continue or terminate pregnancies diagnosed with sex chromosome abnormalities by severity of prognosis, socio-economic level and sex of the fetus. *American Journal of Human Genetics*, **39**, 183A.

Tyler, A., Quarrell, O.J.W., Lazarou, L.P. *et al.* (1990) Exclusion testing in pregnancy for Huntington's disease. *Journal of Medical Genetics*, **27**, 488–495.

Verp, M.S., Bombard, A.T., Simpson, J.L. *et al.* (1988) Parental decision following prenatal diagnosis of fetal chromosome anomalies. *American Journal of Medical Genetics*, **29**, 613–622.

Verschraegen-Spae, M.R.,Van Roy, N., De Perdigo, A. *et al.* (1993) Molecular cytogenetic characterization of marker chromosomes found at prenatal diagnosis. *Prenatal Diagnosis*, **13**, 385–394.

Vleck, C. (1987) Risk assessment, risk perception and decision making about courses of action involving genetic risk: an overview of concepts and methods, in *Genetic Risk, Risk Perception and Decision Making*, (eds G. Evers-Kiebooms, J. Cassiman, H. Van den Berghe and G. d'Ydewalle), Wiley-Liss for the National Foundation–March of Dimes, New York, pp. 209-225.

Warburton, D. (1991) *De novo* balanced chromosome rearrangements and extra marker chromosomes identified at prenatal diagnosis: clinical significance and distribution of breakpoints. *American Journal of Human Genetics*, **49**, 995–1013.

Zarin, D.A. and Pauker, S.G. (1984) Decision analysis as a basis for medical decision making: the tree of Hippocrates. *Journal of Medicine and Philosophy*, **9**, 181–213.

7

The sonographer's dilemma

Jean Hollingsworth

Modern obstetric practice includes ultrasound scans as part of the antenatal care programme offered to the pregnant woman. When this facility was introduced into the obstetric care plan it was soon realized that there were insufficient numbers of medical staff to undertake the volume of work required to satisfy the demand. This role was extended to non-medical staff and soon this group were providing the majority of the obstetric ultrasound service (Royal College of Obstetricians and Gynaecologists, 1984). It was during these formative years that a number of constraints were placed upon the non-medical practitioners, particularly relating to the communication by the radiographer of the result of the scan to the pregnant woman if a problem was identified. Today the culture of the relationship between patients and professionals has altered and pregnant women have access to a wide range of information related to their pregnancies. This information can be explicit when dealing with ultrasound scans. As the technology improves and the knowledge base expands expectations about this aspect of care can be extremely high. However, differences in working practice of the various professionals now involved in obstetric ultrasound may affect direct communication of the scan result when abnormality is suspected. These constraints, together with other factors which affect communication between sonographer and patient are covered in this chapter.

Groups who support women who have experienced pregnancy loss or fetal abnormalities report that there is often a problem with communication related to the initial scan (Stillbirth and Neonatal Death Society, 1991). Many women were not happy with what had or had not been said, how the information was given and when. There was a perceived lack of awareness of the needs of pregnant women when confronted with distressing news.

These patient indictments do not rest easily with the sonographers who seek to carry out their duties to the best of their abilities within the framework of constraints they encounter daily. What can be done to alleviate this situation so that the sonographers are able to practise in a less restrictive environment and women faced with a problem can be assured that information will be offered in an overt, not covert, manner?

REMOVING THE CONSTRAINTS OF PROFESSIONAL DOGMA

Many different groups of people, medical and non-medical, provide obstetric ultrasound services. Midwives, cardiac technicians, physics technicians, radiographers, radiologists, obstetricians, general practitioners, any one with a scientific or hospital qualification. Some of these groups will undertake a formal period of ultrasound training related to general or speciality subjects and may or may not obtain a formal qualification as a result. Others only attend *ad hoc* courses or rely on variable in-service training programmes to be able to conduct, interpret and assess ultrasound examinations. The possession of a recognized ultrasound qualification does not eliminate the constraint of communication of results by particular groups of sonographers. Different professional groups are regulated in their working practices by professional codes of conduct and practice of their particular groups.

The largest of the groups are the radiographers, the majority of whom will have had recognized formal training and be in possession of an ultrasound qualification. However, this particular group of sonographers is governed not only by their own professional body's rules and regulations, but also by what individual clinical heads of departments perceive is right and correct in terms of patient information according to their own codes of practice and conduct. This of course opens up a Pandora's box as many enlightened clinicians give support to non-medical practitioners divulging ultrasound results while others, with their heads in the sand, still insist on more formal and dated methods of communication, complicating further the role of the sonographer in the communication mechanisms. They argue that non-medical sonographers do not have the necessary background in terms of medical training and this might result in the incorrect information being given to the patient, which could have medico-legal consequences. However, sonographers are often more qualified and capable in the analysis of the ultrasound images than members of the various professional bodies who deem it necessary to control their communication.

The role of sonographers in many clinical scenarios is to provide technical information to the appropriate clinician so that the outcome may be judged. This is an archaic view associated with the radiographer's role in providing hard copy so that radiologists may diagnose, prognose and report the findings. Ultrasound examinations today are conducted in real time and it is the person who carries out the scan who is best placed to judge whether a problem is present or not because hard copy ultrasound images do not always reflect what has been identified in real time. Final diagnosis and management must, of course, remain with the medical staff.

It is anathema to radiographers, who are formally trained for a considerable period of time and as a rule hold a recognized qualification, that they, as a group, are the most constrained in terms of communicating the results to the patient. The constraint is imposed by other professionals who may not be as experienced in interpretation and assessment of the obstetric ultrasound scan or even hold a recognized ultrasound qualification. This has the effect of devaluing the sonographer within the professional community where great personal efforts have been made to be accepted as creditable in particular areas. This problem has been addressed by the introduction of schemes of work by the radiographers' professional body. These schemes are meant to alleviate this dilemma by tailoring protocols to suit differing situations. These protocols deal not only with technique but also with how to deal effectively in a standardized way with any situation that may arise. Heavily weighted in the agreed work schemes are the sonographer's recognitions of limitations of knowledge, expertise and training relative to the individual. These state that any radiographer working in obstetric ultrasound must be expert technically and have a wide range of communication skills (Society and College of Radiographers, 1988). No other group, trained or not, is required to comply with similar codes.

IMPROVING THE PERSONAL COMMUNICATION SKILLS OF THE
SONOGRAPHER

Understanding the ultrasound image is necessary if an explanation is to be offered to a woman, but it is not sufficient. The ability of the sonographer to communicate with the woman will be affected not only by professional constraints but also by interpersonal skills.

Some people are able to deal effectively with certain situations naturally, while others are unable to cope. Allowing for all the variations of skill mix, whether trained or not, it will be the attitude of the practitioner towards the woman that will be remembered retrospectively, particularly if the outcome of the pregnancy is poor. This attitude may depend on the sonographer's underlying personality; however, personality can be influenced temporarily or permanently by factors that may be uncontrollable. Many of the sonographers will have had personal or indirect experiences similar to the woman being scanned and these memories may override normal thought processes. A pregnant sonographer or one who is unsuccessfully trying to become pregnant or who has recently lost a pregnancy may be particularly vulnerable. A caring approach from the sonographer will perhaps be the redeeming feature in terms of how the mother is handled, but at what cost to the sonographer? (Ursing and Jorgensen, 1992.)

The type of abnormality that is discovered may determine the way a particular sonographer will react. The following list is by no means comprehensive but serves to highlight the more common problems that may be encountered during a routine obstetric scan:

- fetal death;
- gross structural problems;
- discrete ultrasound markers that may be associated with chromosomal abnormalities but may be transient;
- suspicion of an abnormality but with no concrete evidence;
- confirmation of a problem in a high risk patient;
- multiple pregnancy either expected or unexpected, with suspected abnormality in one or more babies;
- dating for termination of pregnancy.

Abnormalities can be measured quite clearly and concisely in the presence of confirmed pathology but are more difficult to define when dealing with the related ultrasound appearances. Whether equivocal or unequivocal, the ultrasound findings may cause the sonographer considerable dilemmas. Some of these have already been dealt with in terms of the constraints of practice for whatever reason. Here the dilemma to be addressed is the personal effect on the practitioner in the event of the unexpected abnormality and how he/she comes to terms with the situation.

If fetal death is unequivocal then the news to the prospective parent, when conveyed, will be devastating. The sonographer will be thinking about how to reveal this news while still scanning to obtain as much information as possible in order to assist clinical management.

Gross structural defects in the baby may or may not be easily identified and in all of the obstetric scanning scenarios the expectations of an accurate result are incredibly high. The findings will usually require further evaluation to confirm the diagnosis and prognosis. The practitioner will constantly be appraising the situation while scanning and endeavouring to relay the result to the woman in the best possible way.

Multiple pregnancies are by their nature special but each baby has to be scanned as an individual. The problems are compound in terms of technique alone and the combination of normal and abnormal in multiple pregnancy moves the goalposts yet again.

Some sonographers may cope admirably in all of the above scenarios, others will do better with some than with others and some sonographers are poor communicators even in the absence of any abnormality.

RECOGNIZING THE POTENTIAL PROBLEM OF INTERACTION BETWEEN SONOGRAPHER AND PATIENT

The trust between sonographer and patient is part of the professional duty of every sonographer undertaking a scan, and even with complete strangers the initial communication will help to overcome some of the difficulties that may arise. It is essential that a good rapport is achieved before the scan is commenced. Normal courtesies of introduction and a brief explanation of the examination are usually sufficient. It must be recognized that it is more than likely that the operator and patient will be complete strangers meeting for the first time at what is, to the patient, a very personal and emotional occasion.

Initially all appears well, then a subtle change in facial expression and body attitude, and an intense concentration on the monitor being viewed are perhaps the first indications that the routine scan is not as routine as expected. At least that is what the woman being scanned may perceive. It might be nothing at all, just a particular image giving rise to extra concentration for a second or two. The sonographer is actually re-evaluating the situation, perhaps to reach a decision as to whether there is a problem or not, before offering an explanation. These non-verbal signals are received well in advance of any verbal communications.

So what is the problem about telling the patient the result of her scan? It would appear quite straightforward to explain the ultrasound scan results and this is usually the case when the outcome is good. When there is a problem, professional constraints and personal attributes will affect the way in which the sonographer can handle this delicate and sensitive issue. The interaction between sonographer and patient may be affected by the presence of other people (Winkler and Godwin, 1988). The woman may be accompanied by a variety of combinations of people – husband, partner, children, mother, sister, other relatives or friends. All or any of these combinations will present the sonographer with a different perspective as to how to, first of all, establish a communication system suitable to the presenting situation and, secondly, how to deal with not only the patient but also with any other people that may be present.

No two situations will be identical in all respects. The problem, the sonographer and other conditions may be identical but the pregnant woman and her family will be different, creating a multitude of different levels of interaction dependent upon the expectations of all taking part. It is when an abnormality is detected that the relationship between sonographer and patient will be most vulnerable, more so when constraints of whatever kind are introduced into the equation. In this case both the patient and the sonographer who has discovered the problem may find the exchange unsatisfactory. Faced with constraints limiting what the sonographer can say to the woman, the practitioner may feel compromised, not in control and frustrated. The skill of the practitioner may be able to avert a potentially difficult situation from developing at that particular time, but this usually involves giving the woman unclear information. Subsequently, when presenting for follow-up examination, it will become apparent to the woman that the initial scan must have detected something necessitating the re-scan. It may be argued that this approach has damage limitation if the follow-up scan turns out to be satisfactory, and so it might! However, what happens when, without adequate information, the woman attends for her next scan without her partner and possibly with young children and is confronted with devastating news. Once again pros and cons can be argued as to which mechanism might be best. There will always be disagreement about what is considered best for other people in particular circumstances. If the sonographer has with-held information from the mother, then added to the tally of pressures on the sonographer will be that of guilt. This will affect the interaction between sonographer and patient. Reports from support groups that help women come to terms with what has happened feature this interface as being one of the most difficult to understand, as both the support groups and the women them-selves are at a loss as to why these problems exist (Support After Termination for Fetal Abnormality, 1992).

It is the sonographer who is in the front line when an abnor-mality is first detected and what happens at this interface may be in some ways as destructive to the sonographer as to the person being scanned. It is impossible to standardize codes of behaviour when dealing with human distress, as the whole spec-trum of human emotions from extreme devastation to quiet acceptance may be displayed upon receipt of less than optimal news. This will have a profound effect on the sonographer who will then be expected to erase this incident instantaneously as if nothing untoward had taken place, in order to proceed with the next scan. In a busy clinic the sonographer will be like a cha-meleon changing styles according to the current situation. The next woman's expectations of her scan will be as high as those of the previous patient and this can cause destabilization of interaction between sonographer and patient.

It is also important to recognize the matrix in which sonogra-phers practise. The variable prevailing conditions, workplace, teaching, training and experience will all place varying degrees of constraint that may prevent adequate communication with the woman. Combined with these variables will be the time gap the patient experiences from the initial scan to actually receiving the result, and this may apply to all patients, not just to those with suspected abnormalities. The mechanisms involved here are often associated with the actual location of the obstetric ultrasound service in relation to the clinical support team.

- The whole obstetric unit or just the ultrasound department may be a satellite of the main hospital, either on- or off-site.
- The obstetric service may be geographically distant from the main support services.
- The obstetric service may be incorporated within the general imaging service.

Each of these situations will generate different problems in terms of communication. The skill mix of staff deployed to these various locations will have a direct influence on how communications with women are managed, especially if they are required to attend for another scan in the event of a second opinion being needed. Delays may occur because of the availability of the appropriate person to carry out the follow-up scan and are not deliberate obstacles but rather are related to the available resources. What is of concern in these widely differing conditions is that the constraints placed on the sonographer preventing discussion at the time of scan may cause the patient, through lack of information, to be lulled into a false sense of security with regard to the outcome of her scan. The sonographer is in the unenviable position of having to develop a language that will inform the patient that another scan will be necessary without revealing the nature of the problem. It will depend very much on the individual sonographer how well this method of communication is executed. If this system is to be condoned then it must be seen as not only protecting the patient from information that may generate avoidable anxiety but also as a protection for a sonographer who is unable to deal satisfactorily with this situation.

Consideration must now be given to the way the pregnant woman communicates with the sonographer. The variety of people presenting for a scan at any one time will be unpredictable. For geographical reasons there may be large groups of ethnic minority women whose attitudes and concept of pregnancy are completely different from those of the indigenous population. Language may be a barrier to effective communication and this certainly complicates the interaction between patient and sonographer and of course *vice versa*. In the absence of adequate support in terms of translation, this group of women will be disadvantaged and, even when support is on hand at the time of the scan, it may be difficult to judge what may or may not have been conveyed to the patient. In these situations non-verbal communication may have great value but care must be taken not to send out inappropriate messages. Whether or not pregnant women have difficulty with communication they will want, as far as possible, to be told the truth at the time of the scan and are confused as to why this may not happen.

It would seem that most women would like sonographers to be honest with them about what they see (Support After Termination For Abnormality, 1992) and that some sonographers are not allowed to be honest and others are not personally capable of being honest. Perhaps some clinicians would be more willing to remove constraints and sonographers would be more able to be candid if the sonographers' training programme included basic counselling skills.

While communication is highlighted as an important skill, very little actual training time is dedicated to certain aspects, such as counselling, role play and how to deal with stress. It is expected that the practitioners will learn how to cope in the hard school of knocks. This, of course, is not good enough in the obstetric scenario, as the aspirations of the prospective parents create a very emotional atmosphere. Obstetric sonographers do not need to become counsellors but attention must given to this skill. The ability to use the correct language in times of stress will be a constructive action assisting not only the sonographer but also the patient when normal forms of communication are difficult to conduct. Women themselves need to be made aware of what the ultrasound scan is all about. Many women accept the ultrasound scan as part of the routine antenatal care and may not be aware of the implications. Information leaflets should be available in all obstetric units describing what ultrasound service is offered in that particular unit, when the scan or scans will be scheduled, how long the average scan may take and any preparation that may be necessary. Above all, there should be an explanation that in the majority of cases all will be well but, should a problem present and a rescan be required, then an explanation will be offered as to why another scan is essential. The simple measures described may help to relieve the pressures placed on both practitioner and patient when confronted with a difficult situation.

In conclusion, it has to be recognized that, over the years since the introduction of routine obstetric ultrasound scans, there has been a subtle but progressive change in what is required from this routine scan from both the clinicians managing pregnant women and the women themselves. It needs to be reinforced that this routine scan is now part of the prenatal diagnostic chain and the first link in this chain will probably be the sonographer. Many of the dilemmas discussed in the text are the result of too slow a response to rapidly changing circumstances. If the demands of today's obstetric patient are to be addressed properly, radical changes in terms of professional dogma, training and control over who actually provides this service will be essential. Sonographers, at the sharp end, must come to terms with the dilemmas they face so that in the future a more human side to their relationships with their patients may be encouraged.

REFERENCES

Royal College of Obstetricians and Gynaecologists (1984) *Report of the RCOG Working Party on Routine Ultrasound Examination in Pregnancy*, Royal College of Obstetricians and Gynaecologists, London.

Society and College of Radiographers (1988) *Code of Professional Conduct for Radiographers*, Society and College of Radiographers, London.

Stillbirth and Neonatal Death Society (1991) *Miscarriage, Stillbirth and Neonatal Death. Guidelines for Professionals*, Stillbirth and Neonatal Death Society, London.

Support After Termination For Abnormality (1992) *Guidelines for Ultrasonographers*, Support After Termination for Fetal Abnormality, Rugby, Warwickshire.

Ursing, I. and Jorgensen, C. (1992) Ultrasound screening during pregnancy: psychological strain experienced by the investigating staff. *Ultrasound in Obstetrics and Gynaecology*, **13**, 100–103.

Winkler, F. and Godwin, J. (1988) *Access of Companions to Obstetric Ultrasound Departments: Report of a Survey for the Department of Health and Social Security*, DHSS.

8

Preimplantation diagnosis

H. Glenn Atkinson and Alan Handyside

INTRODUCTION

Over the last 5 years, a new approach to prenatal diagnosis has been developed for couples who are known to be at risk of having children with an inherited disease. This approach, which aims to avoid the possibility of an affected pregnancy completely, is known as preimplantation diagnosis. It involves detecting the underlying genetic defect in eggs and embryos before the pregnancy becomes established at implantation (Handyside, 1992). Clinical experience with preimplantation diagnosis is still very limited. At present, it is only available in a handful of centres worldwide and only small numbers of couples can be offered treatment. Also, the diseases which can be diagnosed represent only a fraction of the diverse chromosomal and single-gene defects which can be identified by conventional approaches. Nevertheless, it is important for couples to be fully informed of the different options available, if not immediately, in the foreseeable future. Here, therefore, we attempt to explain what pre-implantation diagnosis involves from the potential parents' point of view, which conditions it is applicable to, and which couples are likely to benefit. We also make a preliminary assessment of how successful it is and discuss the problems and ethical issues which arise.

WHAT DOES PREIMPLANTATION DIAGNOSIS INVOLVE?

In principle, preimplantation diagnosis is based on the simple strategy of sampling genetic material from eggs or embryos within the first week of their development following fertilization. This material is used to detect whether the genetic defect is present and whether the embryo will be affected by the disease. Unaffected embryos are then transferred to the womb prior to implantation and the establishment of pregnancy. The first problem to be overcome in practice, therefore, is to recover eggs or embryos at these early stages for analysis. One possibility is to gently flush embryos from the womb by irrigating with culture medium at the appropriate time after normal conception (Sauer *et al.*, 1987; Buster *et al.*, 1985). However, only a single embryo in most cases would be recovered and there are worries about potentially affected embryos remaining in the womb and about causing an ectopic pregnancy by flushing an embryo into the fallopian tubes. Hence all attempts at preimplantation diagnosis have so far relied on methods for human *in vitro* fertilization developed for the treatment of infertility.

In vitro fertilization

For *in vitro* fertilization, a woman is induced to produce several eggs in a single reproductive cycle; the eggs are recovered from the follicles in the ovary at the appropriate time and fertilized and cultured for a period in a 'test tube' before being transferred to the womb. Initially, the woman's own reproductive endocrine cycles are suppressed by gonadotrophin releasing hormone agonists which are self-administered at regular intervals over a period of at least 2 weeks by sniffing a nasal spray (Rutherford *et al.*, 1988). When it is confirmed that ovarian activity as measured by oestrogen levels in the blood has been fully suppressed, superovulation is initiated by daily injections of human menopausal gonadotrophin to stimulate the development of multiple follicles. The progress of these follicles is closely monitored by daily measurement of oestrogen in blood samples indicating follicular synthesis and by ultrasound visualization. The dose of human menopausal gonadotrophin is then adjusted accordingly. Once the size of the follicles reaches a minimum diameter and the associated oestrogen level is high enough, final maturation of the eggs is stimulated by the administration of human chorionic gonadotrophin and the eggs are collected about 36 hours later. To do this, the follicles are punctured and the eggs are flushed out through a needle passed through the vaginal

wall under local anaesthetic and guided by ultrasound. The eggs
(at this stage surrounded by cumulus cells from the follicle) are
then cultured for 6 hours before insemination with the partner's
sperm to allow fertilization.

Fertilized embryos are identified the following morning by
removing the cumulus cells and looking for the two nuclei of
the egg and sperm before they coalesce to form a single embryo
nucleus. Embryos are then cultured until the time of transfer.
Embryo transfer is normally carried out on the second or third
day post-insemination by placing the embryos in a fine catheter,
which is carefully threaded through the cervix into the uterus,
and expelling them in a very small amount of medium. Injections
of progesterone followed by pessaries are often used to maintain
the correct hormonal environment to allow implantation of the
embryos to take place within the uterine cavity. A pregnancy
test is carried out 14 days post-insemination by measuring serum
human chorionic gonadotrophin levels which indicate placental
function. If this is positive, a vaginal ultrasound scan is done 14
days later to assess the position of the pregnancy sac. This scan
is repeated 2 weeks later to see how many embryos have
implanted and to examine for the presence of fetal hearts confirming the progress of fetal development.

Egg and embryo biopsy

For genetic analysis of eggs and embryos, at least one cell has
to be removed or biopsied from each of them. Preconception diagnosis is possible for maternal defects by biopsying the tiny polar
body produced during the formation of the egg, which contains
one set of discarded genes (Verlinsky *et al.*, 1990). Examination
of the polar body for the defective gene enables identification of
the gene retained in the egg. The removal of the polar body does
not affect fertilization or the further development of the embryo.
This approach has the advantage that it is ethically more acceptable to some couples, since it only involves manipulation of
gametes and not embryos. However, polar body analysis is not
always informative and no pregnancies have been reported.

The alternative is to biopsy cells from the developing embryo
after fertilization at stages before implantation, i.e. preimplantation diagnosis. Over this period, the fertilized egg divides or
cleaves in half, quarters and eighths and, by the third day post-

insemination, reaches the eight-cell stage. Two or three days later, after further division and organization of the cells, the embryo reaches the blastocyst stage in preparation for implantation between the seventh and tenth day post-insemination. On day 7, the blastocyst averages 125 cells arranged as a hollow ball, with an outer layer of cells which will mainly form the placenta enclosing a smaller cluster of cells from which the fetus itself is derived (Hardy, Handyside and Winston, 1989). Since embryo transfers are not as successful at later stages, embryos are biopsied at about the eight-cell stage on the morning of the third day (Figure 8.1) This then allows 8–12 hours for analysis before selected unaffected embryos are transferred later the same day.

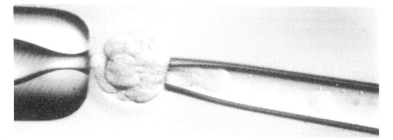

Figure 8.1 Cleavage stage embryo biopsy: a single cell is aspirated from a cleavage stage embryo attached by suction to a holding pipette for genetic analysis. (Photograph taken from video recording.)

Removal of cells at these early stages does not harm the embryo since they have not become specialized (Hardy et al, 1990). In fact, many human embryos have damaged cells and implant and develop normally after transfer following routine *in vitro* fertilization. However, removal of more than two cells is likely to reduce the embryo's ability to implant and develop at all. Nevertheless, couples seeking preimplantation diagnosis need to be counselled that only a small number of children have been born following this procedure and that there is a small but finite risk that unforeseen effects could only become apparent later in their development.

Genetic diagnosis

There are two broad categories of genetic defect causing inherited disease: those which affect chromosomes (the paired structures in the nucleus, one from each parent, on which the genes are arranged); and those which affect only single genes. The restrictions in the number of cells removed by cleavage stage biopsy and the time available for testing severely limit the possibilities for genetic analysis. In fact, preimplantation diagnosis has only been made possible by the recent development of sensitive and rapid methods for analysis of the chromosomes and genes of single cells. Fortunately, the versatility of these methods has opened up the possibility of diagnosing a wide spectrum of different inherited conditions (Table 8.1). So far, however, it has to be stressed that preimplantation diagnosis has only been attempted and pregnancies established in couples at risk of sex-linked diseases (Handyside *et al.*, 1990; Grifo *et al.*, 1992; Griffin *et al.*, 1993), cystic fibrosis (Handyside *et al.*, 1992) Lesch–Nyhan syndrome and Tay–Sachs disease (unpublished data).

Table 8.1 Some common inherited disorders in which preimplantation diagnosis may be feasible

1. Chromosomal defects
Trisomy syndromes
21   Down
18   Edward
13   Patau
XXY   Klinefelter

Monosomy syndrome
XO   Turner

Translocations
eg. 45,XX, t(13;14)

2. Single gene defects
Autosomal dominant
Huntington's disease

Autosomal recessive
Cystic fibrosis
Tay–Sachs
Beta thalassaemia
Sickle cell anaemia

X-linked recessive
Duchenne muscular dystrophy
Haemophilia
Lesch–Nyhan syndrome
X-linked mental retardation

Sex-linked (X-linked) recessive diseases account for 6–7% of single-gene defects and include such prevalent conditions as Duchenne muscular dystrophy, haemophilia and various mental retardation syndromes. Typically, the mother carrying the defect on one of her X chromosomes transmits the defect to half her children. Boys inheriting the defect are affected by the disease because the male Y chromosome inherited from the father does not have the same genes and so there are no copies of the normal gene to compensate. On the other hand, girls inheriting the defect are carriers like their mother but inherit a normal gene on the X chromosome from their fathers and in almost all cases are unaffected. However, they will in turn be at risk of having boys affected by the disease.

Rapid progress is being made to define the exact nature of the genetic defects causing X-linked diseases and single-gene defects in general. However, the location and exact nature of the defect remain unidentified in many cases. In these cases, the alternative option of simply identifying the sex of the conceptus and terminating males with a one in two chance of being affected is all that can be offered even with conventional prenatal diagnosis. The advantage of preimplantation diagnosis is that it is equally applicable to any X-linked recessive disease.

Cystic fibrosis is an ideal candidate for preimplantation diagnosis since, apart from being the most prevalent autosomal recessive disease in the caucasian population, the gene involved has been identified. In most cases, the genetic defect is a small deletion at position delta F508 within the gene (Riordan *et al.*, 1989). Hence in this case, the development of a single strategy enabling detection of this deletion is applicable to a majority of couples at risk of having children with cystic fibrosis. Other examples of diseases caused by a limited number of genetic defects are sickle cell anaemia and Tay–Sachs disease. In both cases, single-cell analysis is now possible and preimplantation diagnosis for Tay–Sachs disease has been successful. For other heterogeneous single-gene defects, however – for example, the haemoglobinopathies – either individual detection strategies will have to be developed for specific families or further research is necessary to enable combined analysis of informative markers.

Further in the future, it may be possible to use techniques for visualizing chromosomes, currently used to identify the sex of embryos with X and Y probes (Griffin *et al.*, 1992), to identify embryos which are likely to spontaneously abort or be affected by a variety of syndromes if they survive to term. The most well known example of these syndromes is trisomy 21 or Down syndrome, caused by inheritance of three copies of the whole, or a critical region, of chromosome 21. Women who have a Down syndrome child are at increased risk of having another. Older women are also at increased risk. However, the risk is much lower than in couples at risk of single-gene defects and screening would probably not be worthwhile. Nevertheless, if detection of abnormal numbers of a combination of chromosomes is practical, as seems possible, it may be beneficial to screen the embryos of older women undergoing *in vitro* fertilization for infertility treatment (Handyside and Delhanty, 1993). Although the frequency is no higher than would be expected after normal conception, it is particularly distressing for a couple to achieve a much wanted pregnancy only to have a baby affected by a chromosomal abnormality. Screening for chromosome abnormalities may also reduce the frequency of miscarriage which increases significantly in older women.

WHAT ARE THE ADVANTAGES OF PREIMPLANTATION DIAGNOSIS?

The principal advantage of preimplantation diagnosis is that it avoids the possibility of having to terminate a pregnancy diagnosed as affected at later stages of gestation. This is the primary motivation of the majority of couples seeking this form of prenatal screening. Typically, these couples have already had affected children (or otherwise have affected family members) and know at first hand the consequences of the condition. Many of them have been unlucky enough to have had repeated terminations of affected pregnancies. Others have had miscarriages as a result of one of the conventional invasive procedures. Paradoxically, couples having preimplantation diagnosis have to be counselled that a follow-up diagnosis by one of the conventional methods (preferably chorionic villus sampling) is advisable since the accuracy of preimplantation diagnosis has yet to be established clinically. However, several couples who have indicated that they would have a follow-up diagnosis have changed their minds when the woman became pregnant, their negative feelings about these procedures outweighing the fear that the preimplantation diagnosis might have been inaccurate.

Methods for sampling fetal cells after implantation involve either amniocentesis in the late first or second trimester or chorionic villus sampling in the first trimester. These procedures are not without risk to the pregnancy, and after them the couple face an agonizing wait for results which may take up to 3 weeks in the case of amniocentesis samples or 5–10 days for a chorionic villus sampling specimen. If the fetus is then found to be affected, the couple must decide whether or not to have a termination of pregnancy. This is with the full knowledge that there is a developing fetus within the woman's womb which has the ability to develop into a human being if allowed to do so. They will obviously have considered this option before having the test, otherwise they would not have accepted prenatal diagnosis. However, a decision made rationally when not pregnant may not seem as clear-cut when the pregnancy has been achieved.

The decision to have an invasive procedure with all its possible sequelae is made all the more difficult with advancing maternal age. Many couples opting for prenatal diagnosis for inherited disease have one affected child. This often means that they will delay trying for a further pregnancy either because they are afraid of the consequences of such a pregnancy or because they wish to make sure that they can adequately cope emotionally and physically with another child. It has to be remembered that going through a pregnancy, birth and caring for a neonate is not easy at the best of times but is extremely difficult when looking after another physically or mentally handicapped child who may be extremely demanding. Once the difficult decision to try for a further pregnancy has been made, the pressure to keep any such pregnancy is great and thus the temptation not to have a test which will endanger it is considerable.

Having opted for prenatal testing, diagnosis of an affected fetus and any subsequent termination of pregnancy must be traumatic psychologically and often physically. It can be such a harrowing and distressing experience that some couples remain voluntarily infertile rather than face the same scenario in a subsequent pregnancy. The motivation, even for repeated attempts at preimplantation diagnosis, is often therefore very high.

Another unanticipated advantage of preimplantation diagnosis, especially for couples with a long history of attempts with conventional approaches, is that the period of trying for an unaffected pregnancy is likely to be relatively short. *In vitro* fertilization pregnancy rates are not high and there is much research into improving the viability and selection of embryos. However, in experienced centres rates are now about one in three embryo transfers. At Hammersmith Hospital in the period 1989 to 1990, the clinical pregnancy rate as measured by the presence of a fetal heart on the ultrasound examination was 34% of those couples who achieved an embryo transfer (Hardy, 1993). The success rate for patients undergoing *in vitro* fertilization for preimplantation diagnosis is currently somewhat lower at 25% per transfer (Handyside *et al.*, 1992). However, this is at least partly explained by the inefficiency of some of the early developmental detection methods used which resulted in failure to identify unaffected embryos for transfer. Nevertheless, pregnancy rates with these predominantly fertile couples seem likely to be similar to those with infertile couples.

Couples having this treatment must therefore be counselled that a pregnancy is only likely to occur in one out of every four cycles performed. This is often quite difficult for a fertile couple to come to terms with. Infertile couples are used to reproductive failure and have, in the main, accepted the difficulties they will face to achieve a pregnancy. For them, *in vitro* fertilization is a lifeline which offers some hope where none existed previously. For the fertile couple undergoing *in vitro* fertilization for preimplantation diagnosis, it seems that *in vitro* fertilization may be reducing their chances of achieving a pregnancy. However, we know that only 80% of previously fertile couples will get pregnant within one year of trying – equivalent to a 7% chance of conceiving per cycle. When the chances of natural conception are pointed out to a couple, they may realize that *in vitro* fertilization has a reasonable success rate in comparison.

Pregnancy rates for *in vitro* fertilization are directly related to the number of eggs obtained, the number fertilized and the number of embryos transferred to the uterus (Hillier *et al.*, 1985). Therefore, the pregnancy rate for patients undergoing *in vitro* fertilization for preimplantation diagnosis would be increased if more embryos were transferred. However, we would be doing the couple who have an affected child to look after a great disservice if, in the pursuit of an increased pregnancy rate, the couples were exposed to the stress of a high order multiple pregnancy. It would be almost as much of a tragedy giving a couple triplets as it would be giving them an affected child. This is true not only because of the severe effects on a family of the sudden arrival of three siblings but also because the triplets are likely to be premature. In a recent series of multiple births, the average duration of triplet pregnancy was 31 weeks (unpublished data). Triplets often need an initial period in hospital followed by intensive home therapy adding to the strain on the family unit. Also, miscarriage is more frequent with multiple pregnancy and this will obviously cause great distress after the pregnancy was achieved as a result of such intensive therapy.

With infertile women, transfer of only one embryo reduces the chance of pregnancy by about half. The aim in preimplantation diagnosis is therefore to identify two unaffected embryos for transfer to achieve an adequate pregnancy rate without risking high order multiple pregnancy. In transferring two embryos, there is a chance of a twin pregnancy, which with infertile couples is approximately 30%. It is thus important for the couple to realize that the transfer of two embryos, if available, is necessary to obtain reasonable pregnancy rates and that they therefore may have a twin pregnancy as a result of the treatment. Fortunately, chorionic villus sampling is possible with twins whereas it would be extremely difficult with higher order pregnancies.

A decision about the suitability of a particular couple for preimplantation diagnosis has to be based first and foremost on whether it is possible to detect the genetic defect they are at risk of transmitting to their children. For X-linked disease, this means confirming with the clinical geneticist referring the patient that the condition will only affect one sex (usually, but not exclusively, boys). Some, like fragile X syndrome, can affect both sexes and these cannot therefore be prevented simply by identifying the sex of embryos. Currently, for cystic fibrosis, it involves confirming that at least one of the partners is carrying the predominant delta F508 deletion that can be detected. Interestingly, with preimplantation diagnosis, if the defect carried by one of the partners has not been identified or cannot be detected, preimplantation diagnosis can still be offered on the basis of avoiding the transfer of those embryos carrying the identifiable defect. Although this means that some of the embryos not transferred will be unaffected carriers and by the same token some of those transferred will be carriers, this is acceptable to most couples. In contrast, if the diagnosis were to be performed on the same basis at later stages, the termination of a fetus with an equal chance of being affected or simply carrying the defect would be less acceptable.

The reproductive status of the couple is an equally important clinical consideration and needs careful assessment when couples who might be suitable for preimplantation diagnosis are first examined. Uppermost amongst these considerations is whether the techniques involved in *in vitro* fertilization are likely to be successful. This primarily depends on the age of the woman. As maternal age increases it becomes increasingly difficult to achieve adequate superovulation and recover sufficient numbers of eggs. It is especially important for preimplantation diagnosis to obtain as many eggs as possible as some embryos may be excluded from transfer after failures of embryo biopsy or diagnosis. As the pregnancy rate is reduced in women undergoing *in vitro* fertilization over the age of 40, it is probably not prudent to undertake this procedure in women of this age. This is a paradox in itself, as mentioned previously, because older women are precisely those who may be less likely to take up conventional prenatal diagnosis when it is offered.

Some couples seeking preimplantation diagnosis are infertile. In some of these cases, this is because the women have previously opted for tubal sterilization to avoid having another affected child and because they do not wish to go through conventional prenatal diagnosis. In other cases, it is simply coincidental. Infertility is a common condition affecting about 15–20% of couples. For some of these patients, *in vitro* fertilization may be the only way to establish a pregnancy and for this reason they are often desperate for a pregnancy. In a recent case, a couple at risk of having boys with haemophilia had five embryos identified as males but with two others the identification failed. The couple were so desperate for a pregnancy they insisted on having embryos transferred but were persuaded to have those of unknown sex in the hope that there was an increased chance they were female and would be unaffected. (Any embryos resulting from *in vitro* fertilization treatment are the property of the couple by law.) They were fully aware that the embryos could be male, with a one in two chance of being affected. However, the woman had gross tubal disease and further attempts were out of the question because both partners were unemployed and could not afford the incidental expenses involved in travelling to the clinic. They therefore felt that this was their only realistic chance of having a child. The woman became pregnant and subsequently delivered an affected male.

This example highlights the necessity of adequately counselling couples about the chances of not being able to transfer any embryos in the unlikely event that they are all diagnosed as affected or because of failure of the diagnosis. It is, however, easy to agree with this in a reasoned discussion hoping that it will not happen. It is much more difficult when faced with the situation in real life. It is important for the clinician involved in assessing suitability for this technique to realize the possible consequences for all the participants, not only the potential mother but also her partner, any affected child they may already have and any unborn child yet to be. It is important to let each partner air his/her feelings about any aspect of the *in vitro* fertilization cycle, the diagnosis and subsequent pregnancy. In a minority of cases, it has become apparent that one partner is not entirely sure about or happy with the procedure. In this case, the couple should be encouraged to talk about their fears and not to go ahead until both are happy.

From the couple's point of view, preimplantation diagnosis, although offering the possibility of avoiding a termination of pregnancy, nevertheless requires a considerable commitment and is not without its own physical, psychological and financial costs. Because this technique is limited to a very few clinics (and is likely to remain so for the foreseeable future), the first problem is often that couples have to travel long distances and during treatment have to stay close to the clinic for several weeks. Another problem is the limited number of cases being carried out at this early stage. There is generally a long delay between the initial assessment and the first treatment cycle. *In vitro* fertilization and preimplantation diagnosis are complex procedures each involving several stages any one of which, if not optimal, will prejudice the outcome. Because there are many stages at which the treatment and diagnosis can fail it is important that the potential parents are aware of these possibilities before they start the treatment.

The couples also need to be counselled about potential medical risks. The process of ovulation induction is achieved using human menopausal gonadotrophin. This is a powerful drug and its effects have to be monitored closely with frequent blood tests and vaginal scans. In rare cases, hyperstimulation syndrome can occur in which the ovary becomes increasingly enlarged by multiple follicles. This can lead to ascites, dehydration, haemo-concentration and eventually renal failure if not monitored. Most cases of this condition are mild and respond to rest and conserva-tive management. However, it may mean a hospital admission and possibly a prolonged period of inactivity. It is particularly important to avoid this condition in women undergoing *in vitro* fertilization for preimplantation diagnosis as the prolonged hos-pital inpatient treatment and debilitation it can cause would be especially distressing if the patient already has an affected child to look after.

As a result of the degree of monitoring which is necessary, involving multiple trips to hospital, daily injections, etc., an *in vitro* fertilization cycle which is progressing normally involves a great deal of commitment. This is often difficult to give when nursing a child with a debilitating illness. Occasionally, super-ovulation may not be adequate. Obtaining enough eggs is especially important for preimplantation diagnosis since the number of embryos available for biopsy must be maximized. If there are insufficient follicles, a cycle may have to be abandoned and treatment restarted on a higher dose of human menopausal gonadotrophin. This can further add to the emotional and physi-cal stress, the patients often feeling that they have had all the treatment involved in a cycle for nothing. It is again necessary to inform patients that there is a chance that this may occur. Although the majority of couples undergoing preimplantation diagnosis are not infertile, there is no evidence from the data available that superovulation with the regimes we use is any easier or more predictable than in infertile patients. If a second cycle is necessary it is generally easier to predict the response and, possibly for this reason, second cycles tend to be more successful in terms of generating follicles and producing several eggs.

Finally, assisted reproduction can offer couples carrying gen-etic defects other alternatives – in particular the use of donor gametes. However, these options are generally less attractive to couples since they have often already expended considerable time and resources in attempts to have their own children. Egg donation involves eggs being recovered from a parous woman donor without any obvious history of genetic disease transmission, fertilization with the partner's sperm and transfer to the woman at risk of transmitting a genetic disease. This may be the only course of action for some couples to achieve a healthy pregnancy because the nature of the genetic defect which they carry is unknown. Couples who undertake this course of action, however, must realize the implications of using donor gametes. For example, the lack of a genetic link with the woman recipient may affect bonding, maternal and paternal feelings and cause stress within the family unit. There is a shortage of patients willing to donate their eggs and a great temptation to use donors who are related or known to the patient. This can cause further problems as to feelings of ownership of the resulting child, jealousies and conflicts between the genetic mother and the mother who gave birth to the child and even their related spouses. The couple must decide whether they will tell any resulting child its parentage. These issues are different from those arising from prenatal or preimplantation diagnosis and formal counselling about them would be needed to reassure all concerned, including the couple and medical personnel, that everybody understands the implications of such an action.

ETHICAL AND LEGAL ASPECTS

The ethical issues raised by preimplantation diagnosis as distinct from conventional methods at later stages of gestation are those concerned, first, with the manipulation of human preimplantation embryos and second, with the use of this approach to screen for genetic defects that would not justify terminating established pregnancies. Ethical objections to the manipulation of human preimplantation embryos are generally based on the view that there is, in principle, no difference between an eight-cell embryo and, for example, a mid-gestation fetus or a child. They are all human individuals and, since informed consent is not possible, should not be interfered with. On this basis, terminating an affected pregnancy halfway through the pregnancy is no more or less acceptable than discarding affected preimplantation embryos. The opposing view draws a sharp distinction between these stages of a human being's development and consequently argues that the ethical constraints are different at each stage. In this case, manipulation of early embryos to remove cells for genetic analysis is acceptable and some would argue that discarding affected embryos is preferable to termination at later stages. Even after normal conception with fertile couples, it is known that many fertilized embryos are lost before implantation often because they have gross genetic, usually chromosomal, defects (Burgoyne, Holland and Stephens, 1991).

Other ethical issues arise out of the possibility that preimplantation diagnosis might be used to screen for genetic characteristics associated with only mild non-life-threatening conditions or with physical characteristics. In these cases, the principle that the couple has the right to choose prenatal screening may still be a sufficient safeguard. After all, a couple is unlikely to elect for *in vitro* fertilization and preimplantation diagnosis unless they feel strongly about the effects of any condition and often know at first hand exactly what is involved because they already have affected children or relatives. Of more concern is the identification of single genes segregating in families that predispose to cancer or heart disease. With so much effort worldwide directed towards mapping the human genome, fears have been expressed about the use of preimplantation diagnosis for 'designer babies'. This is not a realistic prospect, since it overlooks the fact that even with complete knowledge of the human genome, we would only be able to identify embryos with the desired characteristics if the parents had passed on the right combination of genes anyway.

Many clinics are now considering offering preimplantation diagnosis and will be starting their own programmes over the next few years. In the United Kingdom, there is now legislation which regulates the use of any procedure involving human fertilization and embryo manipulation, including preimplantation diagnosis. The alteration of an embryo's genes, for example, even for gene therapy, or the cloning of embryos is illegal. In addition, all *in vitro* fertilization clinics have to be licensed by a government-appointed authority with both specialist and non-specialist members. This authority has the power to withhold a licence if a clinic has not demonstrated minimum standards of competence or if the proposed purpose is not considered to be ethically or otherwise justified. For example, it is unlikely that the authority would sanction the identification of an embryo's sex simply to allow couples to choose the sex of their child. It is important that similar initiatives are taken in other countries to ensure that clinics have the necessary expertise to attempt preimplantation diagnosis and prevent its misuse.

HOW WILL PREIMPLANTATION DIAGNOSIS DEVELOP IN THE FUTURE?

The widespread implementation of *in vitro* fertilization for preimplantation diagnosis of inherited disease is likely to depend on several factors, including the pregnancy success rate, the accuracy of the diagnosis and the cost of the treatment. Pregnancy rates following cleavage stage biopsy are encouraging and even suggest that preimplantation diagnosis may have the additional advantage of reducing the time taken to establish a normal pregnancy. Although more than one *in vitro* fertilization cycle may be needed in some cases, this can be accomplished within a few months, whereas some couples try for a normal child with current methods of prenatal diagnosis over a period of years. It is too soon to assess the accuracy of diagnosis and this will vary according to the technique and the particular defect to be identified. Clearly, any diagnosis based on one or a few cells at these early stages of embryonic development is unlikely to be as accurate as diagnosis following amniocentesis, for example, in which many cells shed from the fetus are analysed. A follow-up chorionic villus sampling or amniocentesis may, therefore, always be necessary to confirm the earlier diagnosis. Nevertheless, if preimplantation diagnosis offers a substantial reduction in the likelihood of having to terminate an affected pregnancy, it may still be a more acceptable option for many couples, especially those who have had previous terminations.

Finally, the high cost of *in vitro* fertilization in some countries, for example in the United States, may prevent couples from choosing to have preimplantation diagnosis instead of less expensive alternatives such as chorionic villus sampling. If the problems of uterine lavage can be overcome, however, this relatively non-invasive procedure would revolutionize prospects for the application of preimplantation diagnosis. In this case, embryos could simply be recovered for biopsy by flushing the uterus following normal conception and early development *in vivo* avoiding much of the expense and discomfort of *in vitro* fertilization. However, this technique has not been successful following superovulation and the risks of leaving affected embryos in the uterus or causing ectopic implantations will need to be overcome.

Preimplantation diagnosis provides a valuable alternative for a minority of couples at risk of having children with an inherited disease. It is technically demanding and exploits some of the latest molecular biology methods. However, it should never be forgotten that the reason it has been developed is to help these often desperate couples, and their wellbeing should be paramount at all times. It would be wrong to be seduced by the technical *'tour de force'* if the procedure was unreliable or clinically ineffective. Nevertheless, initial clinical experience suggests that prospects are good and an increasing number of the more frequent diseases should be detectable within the next few years.

REFERENCES

Burgoyne, P.S., Holland, K. and Stephens, R. (1991) Incidence of numerical chromosome anomalies in human pregnancy estimation from induced and spontaneous abortion data. *Human Reproduction*, **6**, 555–565.

Buster, J.E., Bustillo, M., Rodi, I.A. *et al.* (1985) Biologic and morphologic development of donated human ova recovered by non-surgical uterine lavage. *American Journal of Obstetrics and Gynecology*, **153**(21), 1–217.

Griffin, D.K., Wilton, L.J., Handyside, A.H. *et al.* (1992) Dual fluorescent *in situ* hybridisation for simultaneous detection of X and Y chromosome-specific probes for the sexing of human preimplantation embryonic nuclei. *Human Genetics*, **89**, 18–22.

Griffin, D.K., Wilton, L.J., Handyside, A.H. *et al.* (1993) Pregnancies following the diagnosis of sex in preimplantation embryos by fluorescent *in situ* hybridisation. *British Medical Journal*, **306**, 1382.

Grifo, J.A., Tang, Y.X., Cohen, J. *et al.* (1992) Pregnancy after embryo biopsy and co-amplification of DNA from X and Y chromosomes. *Journal of the American Medical Association*, **268**, 727–729.

Handyside, A.H. (1992) Preimplantation diagnosis. *Current Obstetrics and Gynaecology*, **2**, 85–90.

Handyside, A.H. and Delhanty, J.D.A. (1993) Cleavage stage biopsy of human embryos and diagnosis of X-linked recessive disease, in *Preimplantation Diagnosis of Human Genetic Disease*, (ed. R.G. Edwards), Cambridge University Press, Cambridge, pp. 239–270.

Handyside, A.H., Harper, J. and Winston, R.M.L. (1992a) Preliminary evaluation of the use of *in vitro* fertilisation for preimplantation diagnosis of inherited disease (abstract). *Journal of Reproduction and Fertility*, Abstract Series, **10**, 53.

Handyside, A.H., Kontogianni, E.H., Hardy, K. and Winston, R.M. (1990) Pregnancies from biopsied human preimplantation embryos sexed by Y-specific DNA amplification. *Nature*, **344**, 768–770.

Handyside, A.H., Lesko, J.G., Tarin, J.J. *et al.* (1992b) Birth of a normal girl after *in vitro* fertilisation and preimplantation diagnostic testing for cystic fibrosis. *New England Journal of Medicine*, **327**, 905–909.

Hardy, K. (1993). Development of human blastocysts *in vitro*, in *Preimplantation Embryo Development*, (ed. B. Bavister), Springer-Verlag, New York.

Hardy, K., Handyside, A.H. and Winston, R.M. (1989) The human blastocyst: cell number, death and allocation during late preimplantation development *in vitro*. *Development*, **107**, 597–604.

Hardy, K., Martin, K.L., Leese, H.J. *et al.* (1990) Human preimplantation development *in vitro* is not adversely affected by biopsy at the 8-cell stage. *Human Reproduction*, **5**, 708–714.

Hillier, S.G., Afnan, A.M.M., Margara, R.A. and Winston, R.M.L. (1985) Superovulation strategies before *in vitro* fertilisation. *Clinical Obstetrics and Gynaecology*, **12**(3), 687–723.

Riordan, J., Rommen, J.M., Kerem, B-S. *et al.* (1989) Identification of the cystic fibrosis gene: cloning and characterisation of complementary DNA. *Science*, **245**, 1066–1073.

Rutherford, A.J., Subak-Sharpe, R.J., Dawson, K.J. *et al.* (1988) Improvement of *in vitro* fertilisation after treatment with buserilin, an agonist of luteinising hormone releasing hormone. *British Medical Journal*, **296**, 1765–1768.

Sauer, M.V., Bustillo, M., Rodi, I.A. *et al.* (1987) *In vivo* blastocyst production and ovum yield among fertile women. *Human Reproduction*, **2**, 701–703.

Verlinsky, Y., Ginsberg, N., Lifchez, A. *et al.* (1990) Analysis of the first polar body: preconception genetic diagnosis. *Human Reproduction*, **5**, 826–829.

9

Problems surrounding late prenatal diagnosis

Lucy Turner

During the last quarter of a century prenatal diagnostic procedures have developed with a speed and definition previously unimaginable. However, the race for medical and technological perfection has not given equal consideration to the attendant ethical, legal and particularly emotional dilemmas raised by the diagnosis of fetal abnormality, especially when the diagnosis is offered late in the pregnancy. These issues have been explored in previous chapters and it is sufficient to say here that these dilemmas become more demanding in proportion to the term of gestation when diagnosis is made.

All participants in the process of prenatal diagnosis, parents and carers alike, should have a close understanding of these three aspects of prenatal diagnosis, especially when the diagnosis is made after the time of fetal viability which in the United Kingdom is presently defined as 24 weeks (Human Fertilisation and Embryology Act 1990).

THE DECISION

Perhaps one of the most difficult problems faced by prospective parents developing suspicious symptoms late in pregnancy is whether or not to have prenatal diagnostic investigations. At this stage their circle of family and friends are well aware of their impending parenthood, they have been congratulated and have been given gifts for the forthcoming birth; often the nursery has been decorated and the layette bought. The baby has made its presence felt by kicking and moving about, a dramatic reminder that he or she is alive. Now there is some possibility that the longed-for event may not materialize or, if it does, that it will do so in a way vastly different to what they had expected. One part of their consciousness tells them to 'hope for the best' and carry on to delivery without doing anything to disturb their joyful anticipation. The other part insists they should know what is going on in the mother's womb and provide as best they can for the outcome.

Let us now consider how couples come to be in a position necessitating late prenatal diagnosis. Such couples fall into three groups:

- those who discovered 'late' that they were pregnant, such as women who have a contraceptive failure and continue to 'bleed' each month;
- those in whom a suspected abnormality is detected at an anomaly scan at around 19–20 weeks gestation and who are then referred on to a specialist centre for further investigation and counselling, all of which may take some time;
- those in whom clinical appearances such as polyhydramnios or intrauterine growth retardation, late in the second or into the third trimester, lead to the suspicion of an abnormality.

There are many factors which influence the couple's decision about whether or not to have prenatal tests. These include:

- how the couple perceive the size of the risk at the time the suspicion arises and how they saw it before;
- how their options were communicated to them during counselling;
- their previous understanding of the condition being investigated;
- their individual circumstances;
- their spiritual and moral beliefs.

All couples should be counselled at their first meeting regarding the significance of all the tests and the implications of the results if abnormal. At this initial point the couple should be asked to consider their views on termination of pregnancy and these should be clarified before the test is performed.

It is now that considerate and supportive advice is needed to point out the advantages and disadvantages of having the relevant procedures at this late stage. Those counselling them must take account of the cultures, backgrounds and individual inclinations of the parents as well as their level of intelligence and understanding. While presenting the alternatives in an objective, unbiased fashion, they should gear their approach to minimize guilt for whatever decision is reached. The parents should feel that they can make an informed and personally acceptable decision as regards the diagnostic tests and resulting options.

Parents will suffer the emotional stress of considering whether they will abort if their wanted child is diagnosed as abnormal, and should be offered at this prediagnostic stage the services of other appropriate counsellors. Support groups for the suspected anomaly, geneticists and religious advisors may all be called upon. Although time is of the essence at this late stage and test results may take four or five days to become available, provision should be made for this thorough, sensitive and in-depth prediagnostic counselling as a hurried decision may cause regret or trauma subsequent to the procedure and related decisions.

If the option to continue the pregnancy without further investigation is made following in-depth consultation, the level of support must be maintained by all concerned with no hint of recrimination in subsequent discussions. Continuity of care, with the same midwife and obstetrician attending, so that painful histories need not be repeated, give the couple a feeling of security and support despite their decision not to proceed with the suggested further investigation. Once this rapport has been established they should feel less inhibited in asking for further help from the people they have now come to regard as friends as well as professionals.

Parents who continue with such a pregnancy, including those who may be faced with a stillbirth or an infant who dies shortly after birth, should be given the opportunity to discuss with their key workers a very specific birth plan. This plan should incorporate the optimal site for delivery, monitoring during labour, analgesia levels and the support network to be present. If it is suspected that the baby will be stillborn or die shortly after delivery, provision should be made for their minister of religion to be present if desired and for the parents to have time with the dead or dying baby. Sensitive questioning should elucidate their wishes regarding possible funeral arrangements. The above considerations, of course, apply to all parents whether late prenatal diagnosis was accepted or not.

IS LATE SCREENING AND PRENATAL DIAGNOSIS ALWAYS A 'GOOD THING'?

Three main factors influence whether women undergo late prenatal screening and diagnosis: the availability of the test, the experience and attitudes of health professionals and the knowledge and opinions of the women themselves.

Informed uptake and informed refusal of late prenatal diagnosis will be increased by the supplying of more complete information by staff to a better informed client. To achieve this, counselling prior to prenatal diagnosis should include: the purpose of the test and the likelihood that an abnormality will be detected; an explanation of the test procedure, including related risks; the significance of test results both positive and negative; and the options following a positive result so late in pregnancy.

Ultrasound scanning late in the second and into the third trimester of pregnancy is aimed at identifying fetal abnormality in those women at a higher risk and may lead to them being offered further more specific tests. As such, it should be considered a prenatal diagnostic test.

Before embarking on this late ultrasound scan it is crucial that women are adequately informed of the possible findings and the options for further investigation. Health professionals tend to assume that diagnosing fetal abnormality in the later stages of pregnancy provides the best basis for allowing the parents to make a decision regarding the future of the pregnancy. While prenatal diagnosis will provide a much wanted choice for many, for others it will be a choice that they would rather not have to confront.

Jorgensen, Uddenberg and Ursing (1985) looked at women who had a diagnosis of fetal malformation in the 32nd week of pregnancy and found that every woman in the sample, having been told of their fetal abnormality, endured mental instability and trauma during the remainder of their pregnancies. In the event, the imagined 'monster' often turned out to be less horrific than had been anticipated. This also applied to those to whom it had been explained that their child's abnormality was small and correctable.

Therefore, should we all think twice before rushing into performing an ultrasound scan if clinical findings lead us to suspect there may be an underlying anomaly? What do we do if we discover an anomaly? Are we then committing ourselves and the woman to further more invasive investigation at this late stage and subsequently forcing her to make a desperately difficult and often painful decision? These are all questions without a uniformly correct answer, but they should provoke thought in all of us. People may argue that this hypothesis, taken to the extreme, would suggest that simply by making a clinical examination of a pregnant woman we are taking the first step towards perhaps unsought decision making.

On the other hand, our proscription against infanticide reinforces the perceived desirability of prenatal screening: aborting an abnormal fetus is acceptable, allowing newborn babies to die is not (Green, Statham and Snowdon, 1992).

In the United Kingdom, prior to the Human Fertilisation and Embryology Act 1990, the options for a pregnancy following late prenatal diagnosis were very limited. The terms of the previous Abortion Act 1967 allowed no provision for late termination for abnormality, regardless of the severity, thus removing the decision for the parents.

An awesome burden is put on health professionals today. A couple's expectations of a pregnancy and subsequent birth, void of abnormality, allows no room for the unforeseen. Staff too, tend to have unrealistically high expectations and in the unenviable task of conveying bad news are often reticent and feel very inadequate. This is particularly so when fetal abnormality has been diagnosed late in pregnancy, for whatever reason. The staff members then find themselves in a position in which they are going to deliver the blow that will shatter hopes and aspirations for the as yet unborn member of the family.

However, withholding the information is probably not an option and studies have shown that women who learn of fetal abnormality once the child is born may feel cheated and let down by the staff who have withheld the information as a way of extricating themselves from an unpleasant impasse, particularly when many of the women had had suspicions aroused by a change in the medical team's attitude. Most women find any delay in being told the truth, however unpalatable, unacceptable.

CASE STUDIES

Some of the issues discussed so far in this chapter can be illustrated best by looking at individual cases.

Case study 1

Mrs T booked in her third pregnancy at 14 weeks gestation. She had previously delivered a live, healthy boy followed by a spontaneous abortion 2 years later. Both she and her husband were fit and healthy and neither had a family history of congenital abnormality.

When she attended for her anomaly scan at her local hospital, polyhydramnios was noted and an accurate demonstration of a four-chamber view of the fetal heart could not be made. These findings, coupled with her low maternal serum alpha fetoprotein, raised the possibility of a chromosomal abnormality and the couple were referred to a fetal medicine unit at another hospital. A scan in the unit confirmed polyhydramnios and demonstrated a short femur, possible micrognathia and an abnormal four-chamber view of the fetal heart. Mrs T was counselled regarding the high risk of chromosome abnormality and prenatal diagnosis was offered. Mrs T naturally wished to discuss the findings and the options with her husband.

The couple returned to the fetal medicine unit 5 days later for further counselling and another scan. At this time additional abnormalities were noted, all of which are associated with trisomy 18. The couple accepted the offer of fetal blood sampling and this was performed on the same day as the pregnancy was by then in its 25th week. The karyotype confirmed the suspicion of trisomy 18.

The couple were devastated and found it impossible to make any kind of decision at that time. They were comforted by staff and the options for the pregnancy were sensitively explained. They left the unit to go home and digest their predicament, somewhat comforted by being able to call key workers on the unit for further advice at any time.

Mrs T did call her key worker on several occasions over the ensuing couple of days to voice her anxieties. She felt the only real option for her and her family was to terminate the pregnancy but was finding it impossible to make the appointment to come in to do so. She was advised to talk to her minister of religion for spiritual support which she did and found it to be helpful. Following this, and with the help of her key worker, Mrs T set a time limit of a specific day when she would return to the unit with a decision. She had come to realize that if she did not terminate the pregnancy this was in fact a decision to continue and that she therefore could not avoid making a decision.

On the morning of the chosen day Mrs T rang her key worker giving a history of contractions. She was invited to return to the unit where on examination she was found to be in early labour. The decision had been made for her. She delivered a stillborn male infant later on that day.

The following is a verbatim report of how Mrs T felt about the way her pregnancy was handled:

'Before they took blood for the alpha fetoprotein test the reason for the test wasn't explained very well. Down syndrome was mentioned. I felt that by having the test I was doing them a favour. When asked, I replied 'Yes you might as well do it'. I didn't for a minute think of the consequences. It never dawned on me that it would be the start of such a nightmare. When the alpha fetoprotein test was offered I received conflicting advice as to the value of the test from the medical staff, some saying 'have it', others saying that it was a waste of time. This cheesed us off: we didn't know who to believe and this doubt stayed with us throughout the pregnancy, later causing us to doubt the trisomy 18 result we were given. If there was doubt between members of the same medical team as to the worthiness of a test, could they have got our result wrong? Should we therefore continue with the pregnancy and take our chances? Maybe, just maybe, they were wrong.

I think it is very important that mothers are told that one of the main reasons for performing ultrasound scans is to look for fetal abnormality; they are not just to make sure that the baby is alive and growing as I had previously thought.

When they scanned my baby following the alpha fetoprotein test results and the heart defect was discovered I came away from the hospital convinced that my baby had Down syndrome. I felt extremely angry with the hospital. I felt I had been given conflicting advice, not enough information, inadequate explanations, no support and having been given this shattering news I was left to sit out in the corridor alone with not so much as a cup of tea or offer of a phone call to my husband. In such a sensitive situation no one even bothered to say goodbye to me when I left the clinic.

I was referred to another hospital where they had a fetal medicine unit. There was a period of a few days between appointments. When asked afterwards whether I found those days useful in coming to terms with what I had so far been told, the answer was 'no'. I would far rather have gone on to the second hospital that same day if at all possible. I was now hungry for more information.

When I was seen at the fetal medicine unit I felt as if people understood how I felt. I felt 'safe'. Their whole attitude was different. They took the time to sit and talk to us to explain in terms that we understood what the problem was, what it meant for our baby and what other tests could be done to find out more. I felt that I hated the sister and the doctor when they told me that my baby had trisomy 18, although the fact that they were adamant that there was no doubt did help. They were very positive in outlining the situation.

We then had to come to a decision as to what to do. At the back of our minds was still the nagging thought that perhaps they were wrong. Looking back, I don't think we would ever have been able to reach the decision to terminate the pregnancy, and as the sister who helped us at the time kept reminding us, by not making a decision we were in fact making the decision to continue the pregnancy. We obviously talked about it a lot and we both felt deep down that perhaps we had done something to cause this problem, despite being reassured otherwise.

I was so relieved when I went into spontaneous labour: the decision was taken out of my hands. All I wanted now was to get it all over with. I was very scared though, I wondered what I was about to produce, I thought I was about to give birth to a monster.

The staff on the labour ward treated me 'normally', like I was having a live baby. I felt it was all very dignified and I felt in control. They were very encouraging and it helped me a lot. When our baby was born they took him out of the room, cleaned him and dressed him before bringing him back for me to hold. This was a tremendous help. I really don't think I would have coped had they handed me Steven unclean and undressed. His colour shocked me and it would have helped to have been forewarned. The fact that he looked perfect made me angry, as again we both thought, could they have made a mistake?

After discharge from the hospital I felt it was a real anticlimax. We had been showered with so much attention, sympathy and concern leading up to, during and after Steven's birth and suddenly it all stopped. I felt as though I had been abandoned.

When the community midwife called to see me I felt very much as if I was just another client on her list, I didn't feel special and I wanted to feel special. I wanted everyone to realize what I had been through and what I was still going through. The midwife told me that she had had two miscarriages, the last thing I wanted to hear; I wasn't interested in her, I was too involved in my own grief.

I now wish I had spent more time with Steven, seen him more. I also wish there had been some facility to see one of the midwives who had been through it all with me. Either a visit at home, or a number to ring at an allotted time when I knew a midwife was allocated to answering calls from women like me would have been a huge help.'

Case history 2

Another woman, Mrs M, was referred to a fetal medicine unit when a fetal renal tract abnormality was suspected on ultrasound at 31 weeks. She had delivered a normal girl with no complications 4 years previously.

In this pregnancy, she had a normal anomaly scan at 22 weeks gestation, although a low-lying placenta was diagnosed.

The pregnancy progressed without complication until a repeat scan for placental localization revealed the renal anomaly.

The findings were not straightforward and further investigations including karyotyping and amniotic infusion were performed. Mrs M's case was discussed with a paediatric urologist who subsequently also counselled the couple.

The karyotype was normal and Mr and Mrs M were counselled that there was no guarantee about the baby's outcome. They were told that the baby might suffer and die from lung hypoplasia secondary to the lack of amniotic fluid before reaching the paediatricians specializing in renal medicine. They were also told that the baby might also need immediate renal dialysis and possibly a kidney transplant. On the other hand, it was explained that there was a chance that the baby might be well and require minimal treatment. Naturally, the decision about continuing the pregnancy was particularly difficult given the wide spectrum of possible outcomes for their unborn child.

They decided to continue the pregnancy and their son was born by caesarian section at 34 weeks gestation but died 19 hours later in his parents' arms, from lung hypoplasia.

Here Mrs M recalls her feelings and thoughts at and around the time of the prenatal diagnosis being made, the decision making and the eventual outcome.

'I remember wondering why they were sending me to another hospital. Was it because they had a better scanning machine? I was led to believe, or perhaps I wanted to believe, it would be a case of emptying the baby's bladder and deciding on the right time for delivery. I was totally unprepared for what was to come. I never dreamt in a million years that there was something so wrong and that he would die. I thought it was a straightforward, simple problem that would easily be corrected.

I hated the doctor that broke the bad news to us. I felt that she had taken everything away from me. The bottom had fallen out of my world, why me, why now, why wasn't it picked up earlier, why, why, why? I was in a state of shock and total disbelief; I wanted to turn around to find she was talking to someone else.

I now wanted to know everything that could be done, the

investigations, the care after he was delivered, everything. The fact that the doctor had given him such a little chance of survival made me think, 'I will prove you all wrong; he is going to survive.' When we found out that he didn't have Down syndrome and that some of the other results were not as expected and therefore difficult to interpret, I thought, 'I'm not going to write my baby off just because everyone else has', which was how I felt at the time.

For a very short time after hearing the bad news I thought that I didn't want to walk around with what I saw then as a dead baby inside me. When I got home and thought about it, I soon changed my way of thinking and although the sheer horror that something was wrong with my baby had hit me, I thought, 'He's still a feeling little person in there'. I then knew that I would carry on and do everything for him and give him every chance.

I'm glad I knew about his problems before he was born; it didn't cushion the blow, but it would have been worse had I not known. It was very difficult to accept his death when looking at him. He looked so beautiful and perfect.

After his death I only wanted to be with my husband and daughter. I didn't even want my mother. I was finding it difficult enough to cope with my own grief without hers as well. I was so distraught; I felt that I had let both my husband and daughter down.

It is now 3 months ago, and I still have this huge hole that I cannot fill, and finding someone who is willing just to sit and listen to me is so helpful.'

Case history 3

Mrs W (a 30-year-old with one normal son) had an anomaly scan that showed an umbilical cord with two blood vessels and mild polyhydramnios. As a result of these findings she was referred to a fetal medicine unit for a further detailed scan and counselling. This next scan confirmed the presence of a two-vessel cord, but there was now also a suspicion of a claw hand.

She returned again to the fetal medicine unit. The previously diagnosed abnormalities were confirmed and both fetal hands were found to abnormal. Mrs W had attended this appointment alone and was counselled as to the risks of chromosomal abnormality. At this stage the pregnancy had already advanced into the 28th week of gestation. A fetal blood sampling to determine fetal karyotype as quickly as possible was offered but Mrs W declined, not wishing to put the pregnancy at risk, stating she would not terminate even if the results were abnormal. The option of amniocentesis was also offered, carrying less of a risk, but taking longer for the results to become available. This was accepted as she felt it might help her to come to terms with the prospect of giving birth to an abnormal child without the higher risk of the fetal blood sample.

Mrs W then left to go on holiday with her family. While she was away the karyotype results showed trisomy 18. On return from their holiday Mr and Mrs W were invited to return to the fetal medicine unit to hear the results of the karyotype and to discuss the options for the pregnancy. This they did and, naturally devastated, they asked for time to think over the options that had been given to them including that of termination of pregnancy following a lethal injection of potassium chloride into the fetal heart.

They returned 2 days later for further discussion and decided, despite their previous beliefs, to opt for termination of pregnancy preceded by fetocide by potassium chloride.

This was arranged, and was carried out 5 days later at the parents' request when the pregnancy was at 33 weeks gestation.

'I just couldn't believe what I was hearing; my baby that had now been kicking inside me for the best part of 3 months was abnormal. When I agreed to the amniocentesis test I had not really thought that I would find myself in this hellish position; that is why I went for it thinking 'well what will be will be; we'll cope with a handicapped child'.

How wrong I was! Now faced with the grim reality of it all, I soon started to realize that I had started something by having that test that would be extremely difficult to finish.

We had to think of our little boy: was it fair on him? Could he cope, could I cope, could we cope?

We went home to mull over our thoughts, numbed by the news. We knew we had to make a decision and in the not too distant future. The options were all ghastly – to continue on for possibly another 7 or 8 weeks carrying a baby that probably would not survive but, if it did, would be handicapped. The alternative, terminating our baby after the injection that would kill it, was abhorrent. There was no easy way out – that soon became clear – and after two days of agonizing, we decided to end it then and not prolong the torture any longer.

The day that we went to the hospital for the procedure to be carried out haunts me now – the overwhelming guilt I felt for what I was about to do. The room where it all began with the scan and amniocentesis was now witness to the murder, or that is how I perceived it at the time, of my baby. It was so hard to lie there while they did it. I had to hold on to the bed to stop myself jumping off it or shouting at them to stop. Not that that was what I wanted, it was just the guilt I was feeling and whether I would be able to live with it for the rest of my life. They turned the ultrasound screen away from my view, and although I didn't witness my baby's heart stopping the staff's faces said it all – I felt so sorry for them too, what a frightful thing to ask anyone to do.

I don't regret my decision now, a year has past, but the feelings of guilt are no less than they were that dreadful day.'

EFFECTS ON STAFF

We have seen how parents feel, but what about the staff? They are, after all, only human.

Staff often need help in developing their non-verbal communication skills, as it is in this area that bad news is often communicated long before anything is actually said. The parents feel confused and isolated when staff unconsciously talk in medical jargon. Parents with limited intellectual ability or those whose understanding of English is not good may need careful explanation in everyday language and the services of an interpreter if necessary.

Staff are not exempt from feelings and may also share in the parent's grief. Repeated exposure in no way lessens the intense feelings: when fetal abnormality is discovered 'late' in pregnancy, the obstetrician and midwife have also felt the baby kicking when palpating the mother's abdomen, auscultated the fetal heartbeat and watched him or her on the ultrasound scan, thus making the task of assisting the couple in making decisions for the future of their pregnancy more demanding.

Although most couples find comfort in knowing that staff too are sorrowful, others find support in honest dispassionate medical explanations as it helps them to maintain some self control and composure.

There is a crucial difference between terminating a fetus at 12 weeks gestation and terminating a baby at 32 weeks. For, after all, at 32 weeks a terminated pregnancy has the potential of producing a live baby, thus creating a worse scenario for the parents. This then puts the parents and those caring for them in the unenviable position of electing whether to actively kill the baby prior to the induction of labour, thus ensuring no possibility of a severely handicapped baby being born. It would be distressing for the parents and labour ward staff for such a baby to show signs of life, and it would also put the paediatricians in a very difficult situation. Do they resuscitate a baby who supposedly was 'terminated' and who, if resuscitated, might survive with little or no quality of life? This would be quite the opposite to what was intended.

The alternative, killing the baby, is also very painful for the parents and staff carrying out the procedure. It can be achieved by injecting a lethal dose of potassium chloride into the fetal heart. This procedure is generally carried out in fetal medicine units under ultrasound guidance using the same technique as that used for fetal blood sampling. The fact that the process is carried out using ultrasound means that the staff involved witness the life and subsequent death of the baby, as a result of their actions, on the screen. The guilt involved can be overwhelming, despite the decision having not been made lightly and knowing that the decision and its consequences will produce the most acceptable outcome for the parents. It is at times like these that staff need extra support from each other and often from outside agencies or counsellors.

It is vital that the staff who are helping the couple through the decision process are clear about their own feelings surrounding late termination of pregnancy and feel comfortable with these issues. Staff should feel able to turn to each other for support and may benefit from support groups.

In conclusion, late prenatal diagnosis is here to stay because it can be done. It undoubtedly benefits some people, but the emotional cost to both staff and parents should not be underestimated.

REFERENCES

Abortion Act 1967, HMSO, London
Green, J., Statham, H. and Snowdon, C. (1992) Screening for fetal abnormalities: attitudes and experiences, in *Obstetrics in the 1990s: Current controversies*, (eds T. Chard and M.P.M. Richards), MacKeith Press, London.
Human Fertilisation and Embryology Act 1990, HMSO, London.
Jorgensen, C., Uddenberg, N. and Ursing, Z. (1985) Ultrasound diagnosis of fetal malformation in the second trimester: the psychological reactions of the women. *Journal of Psychosomatic Obstetrics and Gynecology*, **4**, 31–40.

FURTHER READING

Borg, S. and Lasker, J. (1982) *When Pregnancy Fails*, Routledge & Kegan Paul, London.
Brock, D.J.H., Rodeck, C.H. and Ferguson, M.A. (1992) *Prenatal Diagnosis and Screening*, Churchill Livingstone, Edinburgh.
Harper, P.S. (1981) *Practical Genetic Counselling*, John Wright, Bristol.
Jolly, J. (1987) *Missed Beginnings – Death Before Life has been Established*, Austin Cornish, in association with the Lisa Sainsbury Foundation, Croydon, Surrey.

10

Problems surrounding selective fetocide

Elizabeth M. Bryan

For the 9000 or so couples in the United Kingdom expecting twins each year, the risk of giving birth to a baby with a congenital anomaly is not only doubled because of the two babies but increased further because the average age of mothers of twins is higher than that of mothers of singletons. Furthermore twins, as such, particularly monozygotic pairs, are at a greater risk of being affected.

MULTIPLE PREGNANCIES

The relative risk of some abnormalities in a multiple pregnancy differs from that in a single pregnancy. For instance, trisomy 21 is less common in twins whereas some neural tube defects are more common. On the other hand, concordance for neural tube defects, even in monozygotic twins, is unusual and Down syndrome, although usually concordant in monozygotic twins, rarely affects both of a dizygotic pair.

With two fetuses the combined risk of at least one being affected is inevitably higher than in a single pregnancy. Some would therefore argue that amniocentesis should be offered to women with multiple pregnancies at a younger age (Rodis *et al.*, 1990). However the results of amniocentesis may present a far greater dilemma for parents of twins than of singletons.

If both babies are normal, the parents can feel reassured. If both are abnormal, it is a tragedy but a decision to terminate the pregnancy is probably no more complicated than with a single child. Indeed, many would feel the decision to be easier in that the burden of two children with very special needs would be even greater. In these circumstances most couples who had actually chosen to have the test done will probably proceed to have the whole pregnancy terminated.

If one baby is normal and the other is abnormal the dilemma can plainly be agonizing. In the past the choice lay between terminating the whole pregnancy or persisting with it knowing that one baby would be handicapped and require special care while the parents were also responding to the healthy child's needs. Many couples who would not hesitate to have a pregnancy terminated for a single abnormal fetus find it difficult to agree when the sacrifice of a normal baby is also involved.

There is another choice, however: selective fetocide. The intrauterine killing of an abnormal fetus in a multiple pregnancy has been performed for a number of anomalies where only one twin is affected, including trisomy 21, Tay–Sachs disease, Hurler syndrome, Turner syndrome, microcephaly, spina bifida, haemophilia, Duchenne muscular dystrophy, epidermolysis bullosa, thalassaemia and cystic fibrosis.

The methods used include injection of air into the umbilical vein of the affected fetus or potassium chloride into the heart. In a few cases the fetus has been removed by hysterotomy. The mother is then spared the psychologically distressing experience of carrying a dead baby. However the risk of precipitating premature labour is considered to be too high by most obstetricians.

The decision to proceed with selective fetocide will partly depend on the severity of the abnormality (and this can be difficult to estimate in conditions with variable degrees of mental retardation such as Turner or Klinefelter syndrome). But it will depend also on whether the child is likely to die at or soon after birth or survive as a burden to him/herself, his/her twin and his/her family, perhaps for many years. A further consideration must of course be the continuing safety of the unaffected twin fetus. An abnormal fetus may actually jeopardize the life of the healthy child, as in cases where an anencephalic fetus causes polyhydramnios and thus induces premature labour. Chorionicity is one other important consideration. Selective fetocide is contraindicated in the two thirds of monozygotic twins who have a monochorionic placenta and therefore a shared circulation. All dizygotic twins and a third of monozygotic twins have dichorionic placentas. For all of these, selective fetocide is technically feasible.

Selective fetocide is a superficially easy solution but may seem bizarre and horrifying to many doctors as well as to parents. Few parents will have even heard of selective fetocide before being faced with the option. Many will be horrified at the concept and the difficulty of coming to terms with these feelings may be harder when relatives, friends and even doctors show their shock, incredulity or revulsion.

Professionals need to be aware of their own complex feelings, before offering guidance or support to others. Many parents have been disconcerted by their doctor's ignorance. Parents may seek the advice and help of their general practitioner, who will almost certainly never have come across such a case before in the practice. Communication between primary and secondary care is vital if the general practitioner who knows the family is to be able to offer long-term support.

A careful explanation to the couple of exactly what is involved in the procedure is all the more important because they are unlikely to find much written information about it. Some mothers have, for instance, been disconcerted by the sudden cessation of movements in one part of their abdomen. The side effects of the sympathomimetic drugs given to prevent the onset of premature labour may be found distressing. It can be very helpful for a couple to meet another couple who have been through the experience.

When parents are offered the option of selective fetocide they must also be told about the potential risks attached to the procedure. These include precipitating an abortion or preterm labour, the introduction of infection and the possibility, however remote, of incorrect selection of the target fetus. Failure to kill the fetus has also been reported. They should also be offered counselling for their bereavement and the assurance that this is available not only during the period immediately after their loss but in the longer term.

It seems that some people who would agree to the termination of a single pregnancy cannot accept selective fetocide either for a congenital anomaly or in order to reduce the number of fetuses (Evans *et al.*, 1991). In addition to the loss of a wanted baby, selective fetocide raises uncomfortable ethical issues and uneasy associations with eugenics (Bryan, Higgins and Harvey, 1991).

For both parents and staff, the termination of a pregnancy, where the fetus dies because it was delivered too soon, may feel easier to accept than selective fetocide. With selective fetocide, it is harder to deceive yourself – the baby is killed in its mother's womb.

In the case of a higher order pregnancy, each baby has the same potential for a normal healthy life and an apparently arbitrary decision on the fate of a precious baby can be very disturbing. Even though the fetus selection is usually made on the grounds of technical accessibility, parents may feel that they are playing God in sacrificing one baby in preference over another. As one mother said, 'How could you say I'll kill him but not her?'. It is therefore all the more necessary to identify and clarify beforehand the emotional issues that are stirred up. Although the surviving fetus should suffer no physical ill effects, the thought of a live baby lying for many weeks by the side of his dead twin can be very distressing. Moreover, when no fetus has actually been expelled, the natural tendency to deny and forget the sad reality becomes much easier and feelings of loss are postponed.

BEREAVEMENT

For many parents the full impact of the bereavement is not felt until the delivery many weeks later of a solitary live baby. This is also when undeniable proof arrives that the couple will not after all enjoy being the parents of twins. Moreover, in contrast to a simple termination, there is a much greater awareness of the baby that might have been because of the presence of the survivor. Furthermore the bereaved parents have the peculiar and painful difficulty of grieving for a lost baby both during the continuing pregnancy and after the live birth.

By the time of the delivery, especially if it is in a different hospital from that which performed the selective fetocide, the mother's carers may have forgotten that it was a twin pregnancy and their consequent failure to respect the dead baby may add to the mother's distress. A follow-up study of the first 12 mothers in the United Kingdom to have a selective fetocide for discordant anomalies in their twins, found that all 12 felt they had made the correct decision but that many thought their loss had been underestimated or even forgotten, and that bereavement support had been inadequate (Bryan, 1989).

When one twin dies and the other survives, not only the bereaved couple but also those who care for them are faced with contradictory emotional processes. The mother's celebration of the birth of the live baby and her increasing emotional commitment to it contrast with the parallel process of sorrowfully coming to terms with the death of the other baby.

The dead baby may at first seem like a fantasy, particularly if the mother did not see it and has no mementoes of its brief existence such as an ultrasound picture. Some mothers deeply regretted that they were not allowed to see the baby after it was delivered, even when the fetus had been dead for some weeks. As one mother said, 'I wanted to know – I kept asking – they wouldn't show it – they just took it away'.

The lack of respect for the fetus has upset many mothers. One was outraged that a post-mortem should have been performed without even a request for her permission. 'How dare he do it without me knowing? As if the baby was nothing to do with me – this was the baby I had been relating to.' Others said that questions about the fetus seemed to be ignored or avoided.

The bereavement was generally felt more deeply by those who had not expected a problem for one of their much-wanted twins and then discovered an anomaly, such as Down syndrome or anencephaly, than by those who had known all along that they might have to lose the entire pregnancy because of a genetic disorder such as cystic fibrosis or haemophilia.

A mother's full commitment is necessary for the effective physical and emotional nurturing of her newborn live baby. The grief work concerning the lost baby may therefore be postponed and if this process of conscious relinquishment is not resumed later it can give rise to the various syndromes of failed mourning (Lewis and Bryan, 1988). In some cases, however, the mother may grieve compulsively for the dead baby and hence reject the live one. Mothers who have lost one of their newborn twins have been shown to have a higher psychiatric morbidity than those who have lost their only child (Rowe *et al.*, 1978).

Because there is still a live baby it is all too common for the relatives, friends and even medical staff to ignore the bereavement. The parents' loss, if acknowledged at all, is usually greatly underestimated. Ill-considered and insensitive remarks such as 'at least you have got one baby' cause much pain and resentment. Parents of twins are often made to feel guilty about their grief, as if they were being ungrateful for the surviving baby (yet which mother of singletons would ever be rebuked for mourning the loss of one of her children?).

Parents are too often discouraged, even overtly, from talking about the dead baby. If mothers are not allowed to do this they may silently idealize the dead baby and be positively alienated from the survivor.

In coming to terms with her loss the mother needs to be able to distinguish clearly the two babies in her mind; otherwise she may think of the survivor, as one mother put it, as 'only half a baby'. Naming the babies can be particularly helpful. It makes it easier for the parents to distinguish the babies in their minds and when they talk about them. For the survivor, later, it is obviously easier if he can refer to his sibling by name. Many parents like to have a funeral service and some form of memorial. One couple whose twins were miscarried at 22 weeks had a memorial service at which the priest baptized the babies 'by intent'.

Even though the babies can hardly look attractive so long after their death, some parents will still wish to have a photograph of them. Clearly the wish should be respected. A photograph of the ultrasound scan showing both babies may also be – or become – a precious tangible reminder and a unique proof to parents that they ever had a multiple pregnancy.

The pride of being an expectant mother, or father, of twins is enormous and the failure to become one is therefore all the greater. Some parents have found it as hard to come to terms with the loss of twin parenthood as they do with the loss of their baby.

THE SURVIVING TWIN

A surviving twin will usually feel the loss of his twin brother or sister far more deeply than the loss of an ordinary sibling. Strangely enough, this may still be so even when one twin has died before or at birth (Woodward, 1988). This may be due to the intrauterine relationship of twins but little is known about this. Nor is there yet any information on the reactions of the surviving twin following selective fetocide.

It is almost certainly better that the survivor be told about his/her twin from the start. There have been many accounts of painful and unexplained feelings of loss experienced by surviving twins who had not been told about their stillborn twin. Many felt a sense of relief when these feelings were finally explained, sometimes many years later.

A child who knows he/she is a twin can be helped to identify and express his/her feelings. The child may be angry with the parents for 'allowing' the baby to die or may feel anger towards the twin for causing so much unhappiness. Later he/she may have to come to terms with a form of survivor-guilt. It is vital that we should learn about the feelings of a survivor of selective fetocide as soon as possible so that more appropriate counselling can be given to both parents and children.

HIGHER ORDER PREGNANCIES

New techniques in the treatment of infertility have resulted in a worrying increase in the number of higher order pregnancies despite the recent limitations, in British law at least, in the number of embryos that may be implanted to a maximum of three. Some parents will choose to have a reduction of a pregnancy of three or more embryos to two by undergoing selective fetocide at the end of the first trimester. Even if this seems to be the best of some painful options, many parents will feel a lasting grief and guilt over the death of one or more potentially healthy children. The surviving child or children may also be emotionally – and understandably – bewildered by the apparent arbitrariness of their own survival.

Whether described as selective fetocide, selective reduction or selective birth, the group of procedures in question is likely to become more generally available and needs the same deep thought and public discussion as the implications and ethics of terminating a single pregnancy.

It is also vital for follow-up studies to be carried out, on the physical and emotional wellbeing of both the parents and the surviving children. The results will not only suggest what support should be provided but may well influence policy on selective fetocide in general. For many couples selective fetocide may be the least painful of the options facing them but they will still need much understanding and support.

REFERENCES

Bryan, E.M. (1989) The response of mothers to selective fetocide. *Ethical Problems in Reproductive Medicine*, **1**, 28–30.

Bryan, E.M., Higgins, R. and Harvey, D. (1991) Ethical dilemmas, in *The Stress of Multiple Births*, (eds E.M. Bryan and D. Harvey), Multiple Births Foundation, London, pp. 35–40.

Evans, M.I., Drugan, A., Bottoms, S.F. *et al.* (1991) Attitudes on the ethics of abortion, sex selection, and selective pregnancy termination among health care professionals, ethicists, and clergy likely to encounter such situations. *American Journal of Obstetrics and Gynecology*, **164**, 1092–1099.

Lewis, E. and Bryan, E.M. (1988) Management of perinatal loss of a twin. *British Medical Journal*, **297**, 1321–1323.

Rodis, J.F., Egan, J.F.X., Craffey, A. *et al.* (1990) Calculated risk of chromosomal abnormalities in twin gestations. *Obstetrics and Gynecology*, **76**, 1037–1041.

Rowe, J., Clyman, R., Green, C. *et al.* (1978) Follow up of families who experience a perinatal death. *Pediatrics*, **62**, 166–170.

Woodward, J. (1988) The bereaved twin. *Acta Geneticae Medicae Gemellologiae*, **37**, 173–180.

11

Parents' reactions to termination of pregnancy for fetal abnormality: from a mother's point of view

Helen Statham

INTRODUCTION

The aim of prenatal diagnosis is to determine whether or not a fetus has an abnormality. Most parents undergoing testing are told that their baby is not affected by the disorders which have been looked for. Parents told that their unborn baby is malformed have a number of options. The main choices are between terminating or continuing the pregnancy, with additional choices for those who continue which may include considering the time, place and method of delivery, treatment and whether or not to keep the child or place him or her for adoption. It is unlikely, however, that prenatal diagnosis would have been resourced in the way it is just to give parents reassurance, or if most parents with an abnormality chose to continue the pregnancy. The 'enormous potential for the avoidance of serious genetic disease and congenital malformation' (Weatherall, 1992) can only be realized in most cases if women who conceive fetuses with such a genetic disease or malformation terminate the pregnancy.

With the large, captive audience of interested professionals that attended the study day which gave rise to this book, I seized upon the opportunity to talk very specifically about aspects of care for those parents who, given a diagnosis of fetal abnormality, do go on to terminate the pregnancy. I raised a number of questions: how should a diagnosis be given; how long should there be between diagnosis and termination?; should the termination happen on a labour or a gynaecology ward?; should parents see, hold, photograph and bury their babies?; what aftercare do parents need?; and how do staff cope with this difficult area of their work?

I could have followed the same format for this chapter and given a checklist of good practice. However, in the preface our editors say: 'the aim of this book is not to pass on a large body of information; it is to make people think about issues which are vital to the emotional health of pregnant women, their partners and families, workers in the maternity services and society as a whole.' The issues of appropriate standards of care for parents at this time are very important, and they are addressed in detail elsewhere (Support After Termination For Abnormality, 1990; Statham, 1992). Here, I would like to explore the attitudes and emotions of both parents and staff to the process of diagnosis, the detection of abnormality and termination of pregnancy. Unless otherwise acknowledged, all quotations are from women who have written to me or to Support After Termination For Abnormality (SATFA) about their experiences.

WHAT IS A TERMINATION FOR ABNORMALITY?

I used to work in a tissue culture laboratory; sometimes we would receive tissue samples from fetuses aborted because they were at risk of having Duchenne muscular dystrophy. We were always quite pleased to be getting samples of fetal tissue, although we usually had a few concerns – would it be in good condition? What time would it eventually arrive? We also used to think how lucky the woman was not to have to give birth to this (possibly) handicapped child.

A few things have changed over the last 10 years. Research into Duchenne is not so dependent on fetal tissue; prenatal diagnosis is more accurate, so fetuses are not often aborted just because they are male. And I gained some insight into how these 'lucky' women had probably felt when, following amniocentesis, my second child was diagnosed as having Down syndrome. I realized then just how completely I had absorbed the existing medical ethos of a termination for abnormality: the baby with the abnormality is the problem, and the problem can be solved by being taken away.

I have argued previously (Statham, 1992) that such a view was understandable: perinatal deaths were not recognized as traumatic even when they occurred in the most narrowly defined perinatal period. Attitudes to abortion were more liberal, the consequences of an early (non-medical) abortion of an unwanted pregnancy were documented and found not to be severe. Attitudes to prenatal diagnosis drew on both of these perspectives as well as being a real alternative for families who knew that a pregnancy had a high risk of resulting in the birth of a handicapped child. The other available options were either risking a pregnancy or restraint from all pregnancies, including those that would result in the birth of a healthy baby.

In only a few minutes, my science-based attitudes to detection and termination of handicapped fetuses were shaken. Immediately my consultant gave me the news, I lost the healthy baby that I and everyone around me had been expecting; that baby was gone, whatever decision I would subsequently make. In choosing to terminate, I experienced a second bereavement, the physical loss of the baby who was not healthy. 'So I have two griefs really: loss of my Down's baby whom I saw on the ultrasound screen and whose heartbeat I heard with Sonicaid, and loss of the fantasy "perfect" baby we all imagine when we're pregnant.' These two losses are united through a third factor, making this bereavement unique: parents choose to cause the loss: 'The pain of loss, and the pain of having to be the one to make the loss, is the hardest thing I ever have or want to have to go through.' A termination for abnormality is not the taking away of a problem; rather it is the process of adjusting to the knowledge that you have a baby who has a problem; making a difficult and painful decision about what to do; and learning to live with the consequences of that decision. The problem for mothers has been to ensure that these aspects of their experience are recognized, while not denying that, usually, it is a choice that they welcome the opportunity to make: 'Every day I say thank God that they do these tests because I don't know what people did years ago' (Rothman, 1986).

WHY DO WOMEN CHOOSE TO HAVE TESTS?

Some would argue that the question 'why do women choose to have tests?' ignores an important issue: many women do not choose tests. Either they are not given the information on which to make a decision or they do not even know they are having a test. Thus women undergo scanning 'aware' that abnormalities can be detected but 'somehow, when you go for a routine scan for size, you can't believe that they'll find something so dreadful'. In a recent study in a London teaching hospital, 27% of women did not know that they had undergone maternal serum screening for neural tube defects (Marteau *et al.*, 1988). We do not know if women who have not made an informed choice are particularly vulnerable when given a diagnosis of abnormality. In a report of the South Wales pilot project of neonatal screening for Duchenne muscular dystrophy (Bradley, Parsons and Clarke, 1993), the family who reacted most adversely to the diagnosis of Duchenne had apparently not been given information about the test and said that they would not have undergone testing if they had been fully informed.

When I wrote: 'It did not occur to me that the amniocentesis was for any other reason than to remove just one of the worries that as a pessimist had haunted me throughout my first, successful pregnancy. Until the birth, I would still worry about all the other problems that could beset my baby but at least I would know that he or she did not have Down's syndrome' (Statham, 1987), 2 weeks after terminating the pregnancy, I wondered: did it mean that I had not understood the reason for the amniocentesis? Had I been peculiarly naive, even stupid, not to have thought more seriously about the possibility of the alternative, and eventual, outcome?

I would argue that of course I knew the reason, my reason, for the test. If I was naive, I was not unusual. There is now evidence from a number of different studies which shows that women undergo tests for reassurance (Farrant, 1985; Green, Statham and Snowdon, 1993; see also Chapter 3). I was embarking upon what Press and Brown (1991) call a 'ritual of reassurance'. 'Once I knew I was not going to miscarry, I stopped worrying' (Statham, 1987). It is usual at this point to contrast women's hopes for reassurance with the alternative view of the service provider, of 'looking for abnormalities'. This is an important distinction, but is it relevant when an abnormality is discovered? Although there is evidence in the studies listed above that women who undergo diagnosis following an adverse screening test result are particularly anxious while awaiting results of the diagnostic test: 'The period of waiting can only be described as a nightmare', I know of no evidence that shows that these women react any differently to women who were not so anxious when given the news that there is an abnormality. The discovery of an abnormality is always devastating.

DIAGNOSIS OF AN ABNORMALITY

Diagnosis of an abnormality is the immediate loss of a healthy baby. For parents, being told that news is just the beginning of a long process. The person breaking that news may wonder whether, as this is probably the most devastating piece of news the parents will ever have been given, it really matters what is said and how? The answer is, quite definitely, yes, it does matter; at the end of the process, the parents will only have memories. They will relive over and over again the words that were used to break the news to them and the way in which they were said; those words are the starting point of the memories (Support After Termination For Abnormality, 1992; Statham and Dimavicius, 1992). I was recently made aware of a different sort of problem that exists around the time of diagnosis: the conflict that is sometimes experienced by those involved in diagnosis. A particularly honest radiologist described her sense of achievement when she spotted something unusual on an ultrasound scan while knowing that, because she had done her job well, the parents were going to be given devastating news.

Rothman (1986) has suggested that pregnancies are becoming 'tentative'; that is, until after appropriate tests have revealed a healthy baby, the mother holds back from relating to her fetus. While this is undoubtedly true for some women, I would argue that the reason they do this is to try to protect themselves from the pain they know will be associated with the news of an abnormal baby, rather than for consumerist reasons. I do not know of any reports where women given a diagnosis of abnormality ever commented that the pregnancy had been in any way tentative, including those in Rothman's book. Is the idea of the tentative pregnancy a luxury afforded retrospectively only to those who get negative results on diagnostic tests?

MAKING A DECISION

'Congenital abnormalities involve parents in exceptional conflict of revulsion and attachment towards the dead baby, towards themselves and each other.' Bourne and Lewis (1984) were describing parents' reactions to the stillbirth of a baby with abnormalities. When the abnormality is diagnosed during pregnancy, parents experience the same conflicts along with the burden of the decision making; such decisions on matters of life and death are usually dealt with by fate or by God. Can the processes of rational decision making, in which the consequences of each of the alternatives are explored, take place when those making the decision are in shock and under pressure to decide quickly? Yet it is essential that parents reach the right decision. We are starting to learn more about the determinants of parents' decisions (Clayton-Smith, Andrews and Donnai, 1989; Drugan *et al.*, 1990; Pryde *et al.*, 1992). Not surprisingly, the major predictor is severity of the abnormality; such a bald statement, however, ignores the pain in reaching such a 'logical' decision.

The front cover of all SATFA newsletters contains a statement: 'The decision to terminate a wanted baby because of fetal abnormality is one made out of care for the unborn child and in consideration of existing family. It is not a decision taken easily or lightly.' There are many conflicts which parents must resolve in reaching their decision: the baby was wanted – 'Our baby boy, wanted so much, already loved so much and for whom we had such expectations' (Statham, 1992) – yet the decision to terminate says that the baby has become unwanted. Judgments are made on the quality of many lives: that of the life of the unborn baby: 'if he survived the birth, it would mean an operation as soon as he was born and a series of operations which were unlikely to be very successful' (Support After Termination For Abnormality 1993); of the baby when he or she becomes older: 'We finally decided that at 41 years old the worst thing for us to do would be to die and leave an adult with a mental age of 6 or less behind to fend for himself'; of existing children: 'a Down's child would never be company for our little boy, and it would be an enormous responsibility to put on his shoulders in later life.' Women seldom mention their own quality of life, yet we all have hopes for our futures. Those of us who intentionally become pregnant recognize some of the demands that parenting will make on us but see a time when those demands will lessen as the child becomes more independent. Mothers of handicapped children will often not experience the independence of their child and the associated independence for themselves. It is not possible for many women to admit to the selfishness implicit in not wanting to accept a child who will never allow you to become an independent being again. The extent to which this has an impact on both the decision making and subsequent guilt which women experience has not been explored. It is however an issue that does arise in a self-help context such as that provided by SATFA; admitting to my own expectations for my life as being one of the reasons contributing to my decision is often the most valuable comment I make to other women talking about their own feelings of guilt about their actions.

It is widely assumed that early terminations of pregnancy are easier for women than later ones; that the distress that women experience is because the baby has been felt moving and has been seen on a scan. There is some evidence that pregnancy loss at later gestations is associated with more persistent distress (Black, 1989), but some of the women who lost the pregnancy early in this study experienced miscarriages without any prenatal diagnosis. Richard *et al.* (1992) found that women terminating a pregnancy following a chorionic villus diagnosis tended to come for fewer follow-up visits than women terminating following later diagnosis, but there is nothing to support the statement that 'dilatation and evacuation is a preferable method for mid-trimester genetic termination of pregnancy' (Shulman *et al.*, 1989). Why do I raise this issue here, in a section on making a decision? If the assertion is true that what makes terminations for abnormality different from other pregnancy losses is the fact that parents make the decision, and that this is the most difficult aspect for parents, we must remember that parents have to make a decision whenever the abnormality is discovered. A woman whose baby was found to have Down syndrome at 12 weeks of pregnancy wrote: 'It may have been early, it certainly is not easy. The decision to terminate may be straightforward, but living with it is possibly the hardest thing a woman and her partner will ever have to do.'

The extent to which parents really do make decisions after a diagnosis has been questioned: it has been argued that there is no choice about termination, either because of direct pressure from doctors or because of indirect pressure from society in not providing adequate facilities for disabled people. The extent of coercion by doctors is unknown but parents often describe their experiences as though they were directed: 'She was very sympathetic but strongly recommended us to consider termination' (Support After Termination For Abnormality, 1993). Other situations in which parents might say they 'had no choice' refer to the fact that their child had a lethal abnormality. Wertz (1993) has examined the arguments that some feminists have made (Lippman, 1991; Rothman, 1986) that society creates needs for women to be mothers of perfect children such that while women think they have choices they are forced into actions which are determined by social class interests and by society's rejections of people with disabilities. Wertz is unsympathetic to these views, believing that parents' preferences for a child who is healthy are quite normal, but says: 'If freedom of choice means absence of legal coercion, a woman carrying a fetus with a severe genetic disorder is free to abort or carry to term. If choice means being able to live with the consequences of this decision, many women may feel that they "have no choice" because the economic and social costs of raising the child could be unbearable.'

Little is known about how parents who do not terminate cope during the remainder of the pregnancy: anecdotal reports (Watkins, 1989; Green, Statham and Snowdon, 1992) refer only to women carrying fetuses with lethal abnormalities. The woman described by Watkins was 'more emotionally intact 3 months later than the majority of women I have seen who have undergone a later termination on genetic grounds, and clearly, neither partner [feels] the guilt that is unfortunately associated with a decision to interrupt a pregnancy'. Guilt is a serious problem for most parents who choose termination, but Iles (1989) has shown that parents who terminate pregnancies for lethal conditions are less emotionally disturbed than when the baby would live. In addition, it is likely that the support given by Watkins to her patient was instrumental in her emotional state and that women who are part of a study, such as that undertaken by Chitty and Campbell (1992), will find participation in the study a major supportive intervention, as found by Neugebauer *et al.* (1992) when interviewing women following miscarriage.

THE TERMINATION

After the shock of a diagnosis and the pain of decision making, going to hospital for the termination can almost be a relief, but only if it happens at the right time, in the right place and if the mother is fully prepared for what will happen to her. We can only be sure that those three criteria are met if someone has developed a relationship with the woman and her partner since the diagnosis, has informed them of the options available and enabled them to make the right choices.

As with all of the issues discussed here, the timing of the termination is a very individual decision. Some women wish to 'get it over with' as soon as possible, others welcome a delay: 'It did give us time to establish beyond doubt that we wanted a termination, it allowed us to grieve quietly together and to make arrangements for our other child.' Most of us make *post hoc* rationalizations that what happened to us was what should have happened but one woman wrote after an admission within 24 hours: 'It seemed humane at the time. Now, looking back, I realize we didn't have time to be fully prepared for what was going to happen, me physically and both of us emotionally and mentally.'

Her preparation was not helped by the registrar who told her the amniocentesis results. Labour was to be induced, it was to be a 'fairly straightforward process' especially as 'the worst part is over now'. She went on to say: 'He must have been told sometime in his career that waiting for the amnio result is agonizing, and if the outcome is a happy one, then it was the worst part'. With the widespread free distribution of the SATFA parents' handbook to all hospitals in England and Wales since 1991 (Support After Termination For Abnormality, 1990), there is little reason why parents should be uninformed and unprepared for labour and delivery of the baby. The handbook offers parents and their supporters a common language to discuss how labour will happen, how long it will take, what sort of pain relief is available. I hope parents never arrive on any ward expecting a 'mini-labour'; surely that phrase could only have been invented by someone who had not been through it: 'Waiting for something to happen was awful, it seemed so pointless to have to go through all the physical and emotional pain knowing the baby was not going to survive' (Support After Termination For Abnormality, 1993).

Hospitals vary in their policies as to where terminations take place. The right place is where there is a private room where the woman and her partner can be given all the practical and emotional support that they need. The carer should be competent in all aspects of delivering tiny babies, some of whom will be obviously malformed; there should be continuity of care with protocols to ensure that someone has discussed seeing the baby, holding the baby, photographs, funerals, post-mortems, possible retention of the placenta. Whether such care can best be provided in a maternity unit or on a gynaecology ward will vary with facilities in different hospitals, with staff expertise and attitudes and, if she is given a choice, with the woman herself.

The events around the point of delivery are worrying for parents and for staff, with unknowns like whether the baby will be born alive and what it will look like. I was only recently made aware of the extent to which midwives fear the delivery of a baby in whom the abnormalities are not as severe as the parents had expected. The delivery of babies who still show signs of life is not a new occurrence: 'He looked so perfect and I held him until his little heart stopped beating' (Support After Termination For Abnormality, 1991). It is an area of increasing concern for staff fearful of post-24-weeks terminations since the original law relating to abortion in the United Kingdom was changed in 1990. Parents worry that the baby they chose to terminate may be rushed to special care. The biggest fear for parents at this time is, however, about what the baby will look like: 'At first I was unsure whether to see him because I didn't want to be left with a horrible picture in my mind as facial abnormalities had been mentioned' (Support After Termination For Abnormality, 1993). It is rare for parents to regret seeing their baby but not rare at all for parents to regret not seeing him or her (Statham, 1992). In some hospitals fetuses are kept for some time after delivery in case parents who have originally declined to see their baby change their minds, although obviously the situation is different if the baby has to have a post-mortem. Any practice such as this, photographing the baby and sensitive and respectful disposal must be encouraged if women are to be spared a lifetime of regret for making a wrong decision at a stressful time.

AFTERWARDS

On going home, women often experience a tremendous feeling of relief immediately after the termination, a sense of having survived. In some places although there is no statutory requirement to provide aftercare, doctors, midwives and health visitors do so, but for the many women who are left alone, there are questions which must be asked: Am I a mother or not? Have I had a baby or not? The answers are confusing: there is no baby; breasts are unexpectedly full of milk. A midwife would come to a woman with the same bodily symptoms of bleeding, lactation and depression, if there was a baby as well. Why not when there is no such baby? The isolation that women have felt throughout the whole process of diagnosis and termination is reinforced by their isolation from carers when discharged from hospital.

There are resource implications of visiting the woman, but would she not have been visited throughout the pregnancy if that had continued and afterwards if the outcome had been normal? Occasionally, midwives will comment that they asked a woman if she would like a visit and the woman said 'no'; it is likely that if they had just visited, they would have been welcomed. At the time when they feel vulnerable but with no self-esteem, women will not feel worthy of a visit in spite of their desperate need for one. Occasionally, contacts are made that are particularly inappropriate, as in the case of a midwife phoning a woman some weeks after the termination to question why she had not been at her antenatal classes which had just started. Examples of similar administrative disasters can be found more often than today's communication channels should allow; it is distressing for parents and staff alike and is an area where simple protocols could be established to ensure that appropriate people are told of events (Support After Termination For Abnormality, 1991). It is especially important that the woman's family doctor and members of her primary health care team are told of all that has happened to her, as they know her family and background and should be able to offer long term support.

Aftercare also means good genetic counselling, post-mortem results and a physical check up for the woman, not in an antenatal clinic. The result of these should be that the parents have all the information they need to make the right decision about another pregnancy. If that pregnancy occurs, it is a very stressful time; those involved in the care of parents at this time should be aware of the significance of particular rooms, particular dates and even particular personnel.

SAFTA – SUPPORT AROUND TERMINATION FOR ABNORMALITY

SATFA is a registered charity which exists to support parents. It supports parents directly by being there to listen and by providing regular newsletters and information specific to their needs. Although it was called Support **After** Termination, many parents made contact before a termination, and even before a diagnosis (Statham and Green, 1993). Because of this, the name has been changed to Support **Around** Termination For Abnormality although the SAFTA acronym remains the same. SATFA is not a substitute for good medical care but rather works with health professionals involved with parents at the time of diagnosis, termination and afterwards to encourage a greater understanding of parents' needs, to promote good practice and to recognize the support needs of staff in this difficult area of their work. For many women, and their partners, sharing their experience is very supportive: 'I would just like to say your book has helped us a great deal and we couldn't have got through it without the support of the nurses. It has also helped me by putting it in writing to someone who understands what we have gone through' (Support After Termination For Abnormality, 1992).

CONCLUSION

The way in which these feelings were slowly recognized by those involved in offering prenatal testing has been described previously (Statham, 1992). Even as early as 1975, Blumberg reported on post-termination depression, guilt because of decision making and loss of self-esteem because of the conception of an abnormal child (Blumberg et al, 1975). Over the next 10 years, further studies confirmed these findings (Donnai, Charles and Harris, 1981; Leschot, Verjaal and Treffers, 1982). Stillbirth, neonatal death and the birth of a handicapped child were increasingly recognized as distressing events for parents, and Lloyd and

Laurence (1985) and Jorgensen, Uddenberg and Ursing (1985) likened the experiences of women undergoing abortion for fetal abnormality to those of women experiencing a perinatal death. Jorgensen added: 'A decisive difference between stillbirth and abortion of a malformed fetus is that in the case of abortion, the parents have actively decided to terminate the pregnancy, thereby causing the death of a living fetus. The fact that the fetus was malformed might result in even stronger self-accusations and feelings of guilt.'

The message of these papers was that parents terminating pregnancies because of abnormality needed support. By 1989, Laurence was suggesting it was unethical to be offering terminations and not to be offering support to go with them to enable the parents to cope with what was now recognized as a distressing event. Coping was never defined, but as a number of authors commented on 'adverse psychiatric sequelae', it could be assumed to be the prevention of such a response. It would be wrong, however, to assume that support will prevent those features of grief which are found with bereavement: anger, sadness, guilt, disbelief, numbness. Support must recognize the event for what it is, a perinatal bereavement; it must enable parents to react to the chosen loss of their malformed baby in ways appropriate for them. Iles (1989), in one of the few prospective studies of women terminating pregnancies following a diagnosis of abnormality, has started to define a 'normal' response: 39% of women interviewed 1 month after termination were psychiatric cases on the Present State Examination. The proportion of 'cases' had dropped (to the 10% found in a general population) at interviews carried out at 6 and 13 months although a number of women were still experiencing anxiety and depression. Iles's results may underestimate the degree of low emotional state that women not in the study might be experiencing since it is likely that the initial interview was a major supportive intervention; a recent study by Neugebauer *et al.* (1992) has shown such an effect on depression levels of women interviewed at various times after a miscarriage.

It is important to define what is normal, because it helps many parents to be told that what they are doing and feeling is normal, and because it enables us to be more clear about what is abnormal. Patterns of grief following a bereavement are widely recognized; a valuable consequence of aftercare may be to reduce particularly unusual grief reactions and to identify those experiencing adverse reactions. I believe that we know enough about what parents need and how parents feel to establish good practice everywhere and thus ensure that for most women the response to their situation is appropriate. I also believe that the time is now right for us to think about which factors contribute to a less appropriate response, so that support is made available for 'at risk' parents. My impression, gained from talking to many parents over the last 6 years, is that the aspects of their lives which seem to make it more difficult for them to come to terms with the consequences of their decision include:

- infertility, either for the terminated pregnancy or subsequently;
- taking a long time to make a decision;
- lack of social support, especially for women who have not revealed what happened;
- problems with the partner;
- not having wanted to be pregnant.

More controlled studies have suggested that length of gestation, social support, immediate post termination response and whether or not the abnormality is lethal are predictive of later responses (Black, 1990; Iles, 1989).

The number of pregnancies in which a fetal abnormality is detected will not decline. As termination becomes more commonplace, the impact on individual parents of the death of their baby and their role in deciding its death must not be forgotten. 'Although I have had an abortion and it was ultimately my choice, I feel that the scrambled conception and trisomy 21 was a cruel blow of fate. After all, when I conceived the child, I was expecting the best Christmas present I have ever had.'

ACKNOWLEDGEMENTS

My views about the issues I have raised here have come from all of the parents and health professionals who have shared ideas and experiences with me over the last 6 years. Many of the contacts have been made through SATFA, but the views expressed here are mine, and do not always reflect those of SATFA.

REFERENCES

Black, R.B. (1989) A 1 and 6 month follow-up of prenatal diagnosis patients who lost pregnancies. *Prenatal Diagnosis*, **9**, 795–804.

Blumberg, B.D., Golbus, M.S. and Hanson, K.H. (1975) The psychological sequelae of abortion performed for a genetic indication. *American Journal of Obstetrics and Gynecology*, **122**, 799–808.

Bourne, S. and Lewis, E. (1984) Pregnancy after stillbirth or neonatal death. *Lancet*, **2**, 31–33.

Bradley, D.M., Parsons, E.P. and Clarke, A.J. (1993) Experience with screening newborns for Duchenne muscular dystrophy in Wales. *British Medical Journal*, **306**, 357–360.

Clayton-Smith, J., Andrews, T. and Donnai, D. (1989) Genetic counselling and parental decisions following antenatal diagnosis of sex chromosome aneuploidies. *Journal of Obstetrics and Gynaecology*, **10**, 5–7.

Chitty, L. and Campbell, S. (1992) Ultrasound screening for fetal abnormalities, in *Prenatal Diagnosis and Screening*, (eds D.J. Brock, C.H. Rodeck and M.A. Ferguson Smith), Churchill Livingstone, Edinburgh, pp. 595–607.

Donnai, P., Charles, N. and Harris, R. (1981) Attitudes of patients after 'genetic' termination of pregnancy. *British Medical Journal*, **282**, 621–622.

Drugan, A., Greb, A., Johnson, M.P. *et al.* (1990) Determinants of parental decisions to abort for chromosome abnormalities. *Prenatal Diagnosis*, **10**, 483–490.

Farrant, W. (1985) 'Who's for amniocentesis?' The politics of prenatal screening, in *The Sexual Politics of Reproduction*, (ed. H. Homans), Gower, London.

Green, J.M., Statham, H. and Snowdon, C. (1992) Screening for fetal abnormalities: attitudes and experiences, in *Obstetrics in the 1990s: Current Controversies*, (eds T. Chard and M.P.M. Richards), McKeith Press, London.

Green, J.M., Statham, H. and Snowdon, C. (1993) *Pregnancy: A Testing Time. Report of the Cambridge Prenatal Screening Study*, Centre for Family Research, University of Cambridge, Cambridge.

Iles, S. (1989) The loss of early pregnancy. *Bailliere's Clinical Obstetrics and Gynaecology*, **3**, 769–790.

Jorgensen, C., Uddenberg, N. and Ursing, Z. (1985) Ultrasound diagnosis of fetal malformation in the second trimester: the psychological reactions of the women. *Journal of Psychosomatic Obstetrics and Gynecology*, **4**, 31–40.

Leschot, N.J. , Verjaal, M. and Treffers, P.E. (1982) Therapeutic abortion on genetic grounds. *Journal of Psychosomatic Obstetrics and Gynecology*, **1–2**, 47–56.

Lippman, A. (1991) Prenatal genetic testing and screening: constructing needs and reinforcing inequities. *American Journal of Law and Medicine*, **17**, 15–50.

Lloyd, J. and Lawrence, K.M. (1985) Sequelae and support after termination of pregnancy for fetal malformation. *British Medical Journal*, **290**, 907–909.

Marteau, T.M., Johnston, M., Plenicar, M. *et al.* (1988) Development of a self-administered questionnaire to measure women's knowledge of prenatal screening and diagnostic tests. *Journal of Psychosomatic Research*, **32**, 403–408.

Neugebauer, R., Kline, J., O'Connor, P. *et al.* (1992) Depressive symptoms in women in the six months after miscarriage. *American Journal of Obstetrics and Gynecology*, **166**, 104–109.

Press, N.A. and Brown, C.H. (1991) *The Normalization of Prenatal Screening: Women's Acquiescence to the Alpha-fetoprotein Blood Test.* Paper presented in Werner-Gren Symposium No. 113 'The Politics of Reproduction', Teresopolis, Brazil.

Pryde, P.G., Isada, N., Hallak, M. *et al.* (1992) Determinants of parental decision to abort or continue after non-aneuploid ultrasound-detected fetal abnormalities. *Journal of Obstetrics and Gynecology*, **80**, 52–56.

Richard, R., Zonder van, H., Verjaal, M. and Leschot, N.J. (1992) *Termination of Pregnancy after First Trimester Chorion Villus Sampling: A Need for Supportive Counselling.* Paper presented to the 3rd European Meeting on Psychosocial Aspects of Genetics, Nottingham.

Rothman, B.K. (1986) *The Tentative Pregnancy: Prenatal Diagnosis and the Future of Motherhood*, Viking Penguin, New York.

Shulman, L.P., Ling, S.W., Myers, C.M. *et al.* (1989) Dilatation and evacuation is a preferable method for mid-trimester genetic termination of pregnancy (letter). *Prenatal Diagnosis*, **9**, 741–742.

Statham, H.E. (1987) Cold comfort. *Guardian*, **24 March**, 26.

Statham, H.E. (1992) Professional understanding and parents' experience of termination, in *Prenatal Diagnosis and Screening*, (eds D.J. Brock, C.H. Rodeck and M.A. Ferguson Smith), Churchill Livingstone, Edinburgh, pp. 697–702.

Statham, H.E. and Dimavicius, J. (1992) How do you give the bad news to parents? *Birth*, **19**, 103–104.

Statham, H. and Green, J.M. (1993) Issues raised by serum screening for Down's Syndrome: some women's experiences. *British Medical Journal* (in press).

Support After Termination For Abnormality (1990) *Support After Termination For Abnormality: A Parents' Handbook*, SATFA, London

Support After Termination For Abnormality (1991) *SATFA News*, **November 1991**.

Support After Termination For Abnormality (1992) *SATFA Guidelines: Ultrasonographers*, SATFA, London.

Support After Termination For Abnormality (1993) *SATFA News*, **February 1993**.

Watkins, D. (1989) An alternative to termination of pregnancy. *Practitioner*, **233**, 990–992.

Weatherall, D.J. (1992) Foreword, in *Prenatal Diagnosis and Screening*, (eds D.J. Brock, C.H. Rodeck and M.A. Ferguson Smith), Churchill Livingstone, Edinburgh.

Wertz, D. (1993) A critique of some feminist challenges to prenatal diagnosis. *Journal of Women's Health*, **2** (in press).

12

Parents' reactions to termination of pregnancy for fetal abnormality: from a father's point of view

Ray D. Hall

A PERSONAL PERSPECTIVE

As the author of this piece I do not bring any professional expertise to the subject. Nor am I drawing on any research that has been undertaken on the experience of fathers who find themselves in this situation; indeed I am not aware that there is very much relevant research. I was the father of a malformed baby that was terminated, and what I have written largely reflects my own experience. Following the termination, my wife Celia and I became involved with Support After Termination For Abnormality (SATFA), a charity which provides support for parents who have had a termination because of an abnormality. This has brought me into contact with a number of men who have talked about their experiences. I have, to a certain extent, been able to draw on what I have heard from others to try to say something of more general interest.

I am sure that there is much that can be said about how men fare when there is a termination for abnormality. I have not attempted to try to cover all the ground, but there were two problems that I experienced that I know have also troubled other fathers. The first arose from trying to cope with the termination, while at the same time giving support to my wife. The second is the reluctance that I, and I suspect many men, feel about discussing the termination or their feelings about what happened.

PROVIDING SUPPORT

The first that I knew of a problem was when Celia called me at work. This was our third child and, like our others, it was a planned pregnancy and we were looking forward to the new baby. Although the pregnancy was not yet halfway through I had already fitted the baby into my picture of the world. Celia had been more uncomfortable this time around, with much stronger bouts of morning sickness, but we had no thought that anything might be wrong with the baby. She had gone to the local hospital for a routine ultrasound scan to check her dates and the baby's development. We were not anxious, and I did not give the possibility of any problem even a passing thought.

As soon as Celia spoke I knew that there was something wrong. It took me a few moments to understand what she was saying. There was something wrong with the shape of our baby's head and Celia would have to have further tests at a hospital with a more sophisticated ultrasound device. We had an appointment in a few days. Nothing was certain but, from what she had seen and the reaction of the hospital staff, Celia was sure that there was a serious problem.

That phone call marked the start of a rush of events and, looking back, set the pattern for the coming weeks. This whole period, from the time of the diagnosis until shortly after the termination, was very intense and difficult for both of us. Finding out that the baby had spina bifida came as a profound shock to both of us. We talked over what we had been told again and again, trying to come to terms with what was happening. Celia was distraught and later with the physical trauma of the termination to recover from she was in a particularly distressed state. I could barely believe what was happening; it all seemed out of focus. But, although I was in a bad way, I felt that Celia's pain and distress was more acute than mine. She had carried the baby and had undergone the termination. It therefore seemed perfectly natural that I should adopt a supportive role and try to help her through what was happening to us. My reaction was reinforced by the idea that as a man I should be strong and provide a shoulder to cry on, and that I should keep a grip on my own emotions.

This is by no means bad. Someone has to take on that role, if for no other reason than to deal with the practical side of life. Celia was in no condition to continue with her teaching job and could not cope with running the home or with our other two children. I had to 'keep the family going' as well as support her emotionally. Taking on those responsibilities while at the same time balancing the demands of a job was very stressful.

It also meant that I made sure I was always at subsequent hospital visits. My initial feeling, on hearing about the results of the ultrasound scan, had been one of guilt. I felt that I should have been there at the hospital. Being present at later visits not only assuaged those feelings but it also helped in understanding the abnormality and what it would mean for our baby if it were born. Seeing our child and the deformity (which in this case was a severe form of spina bifida) confirmed at first hand that there was a problem and gave us the opportunity to talk through its implications with the doctor. In that way we were both in a position to take responsibility for what was happening to us. The burden was shared.

For me, the down side of taking on a strong supportive role was that I felt inhibited about expressing and perhaps even experiencing my own feelings of grief. I submerged my feelings and that was harmful to my emotional wellbeing and also to our relationship. There were days when I was trying to support Celia without 'being there' myself. This, I am afraid, meant that at times I appeared unaffected by what had happened and perhaps uncaring.

I know, from hearing others talk, that I am not the only father that has found himself in this position. Finding a way of handling these situations without falling into this trap is difficult. The force of circumstance and perceptions about how men are supposed to behave are not easy to overcome. I doubt that there is any general answer to this 'problem', but many things can be done to help. Doctors, hospital staff and other professionals can help by their handling of the father. It is natural that the woman is the focus for treatment, attention and sympathy where there is a termination for abnormality, but it is important not to underestimate the impact of these events on men. Discovering that you have fathered a deformed baby, deciding what you should do about it, being present at the termination and seeing the baby born, are as emotionally painful for men as for women.

Couples in our position have a variety of experiences with professionals, some good and some not so good. In our case the sympathy and compassion with which we were treated made a tremendous difference to the way in which we coped at the time, and to how I recovered. The termination itself can be a long and solitary ordeal for the father. I could not share Celia's pain; I tried to give her what support I could but, as she was being treated with painkilling drugs, for much of the time I could do no more than sit there holding her hand. This was a draining experience. The care and support of the nursing staff who, despite being busy delivering healthy babies, still found time to come and talk to me kept me going. Later on we had the help of a midwife who talked to us about the baby after she was born, and about how the deformity would have affected her development. She helped by taking a photograph and giving us the opportunity to touch and hold our daughter. For me those moments are some of my clearest recollections and, because of the compassion we were shown, have been the most helpful in enabling me to come to terms with what happened. It is of course important for a hospital to provide the right treatment, but looking after both the mother's and the father's needs in a sympathetic way is too important to be exaggerated. This kind of event is rare for most people, and it is important to have someone to lead you through it.

Being caught between coping with tragedy and at the same time supporting others is not of course a problem unique to a termination for abnormality: it arises wherever there is grieving within a family or community. Nor is it a problem that faces the man alone. Women also have to balance their own grief against the need to provide support. Such mutual support is a natural part of any close relationship, but I think that circumstances and the traditional 'strong' role that most men still see themselves as having give a different twist to the problem for men.

The dilemma that I found myself in was not of course hard and fast, but it was a tendency which I slowly became aware of and tried to overcome. While my wife needed support and I tried to give it, there were also times when it was important for us to share our grief and those were opportunities for me to bring out those feelings I had submerged. For us, one such moment came when we sat in the car outside the hospital and, having had confirmation of the diagnosis, we both broke down and cried. This brought us closer together. Other times arose when we talked.

TALKING

When we first learnt about the abnormality, talking was not a problem. I may have been in shock, but there was a clear, factual agenda. Relatives, friends, colleagues and others needed to be told what had happened. This can be a strain if the burden is not shared, but the talk is straightforward, if painful. For ourselves, we had to talk about the baby, about what might have caused the abnormality, about what we should do and what was right.... But afterwards, most people, particularly men, seem to find more difficulty, or are more reluctant to talk about what happened and about how they feel about it. You do not want to burden others with this kind of problem, or you do not know how to bring the subject into a conversation, or how others will react if you do. I think everyone who has been through this kind of experience has had those sticky moments when they have talked about what happened and found it a complete conversation-stopper.

There is a danger that, for a while at least, you may convince yourself that you have coped and that you can get on with your life, but I suspect this is rarely right. Fathering a malformed baby and then deciding, out of love, to end that life is a decision that has a deep emotional cost. Looking back I can see that it had effects that lasted for a long time, long after I believed I had got over it. As the months and then years went by, I may not have thought about the baby every day, but the termination put me under stress which affected not only my performance at work but my relationship with my wife and my health. This is, I suspect, a common experience.

Coming to terms with this loss is a matter of grieving and finding a place for these events in your life, and there is no universal answer about how to do this. People are different and have different personal histories. I have, however, been struck by the fact that few men get involved with self-help groups or seem very willing to talk about their experiences. This may have something to do with the male role of being a source of strength or maybe there is some deeper reason to do with the psychology of men that makes them more reluctant to talk. This is not to say that they will not talk in the right circumstances, but they are reluctant. This seems to be a difference in the way that men and women react. From my experience, there seems to be something in the generalization that while women want to talk about what happened, men want to put it behind them and to get on with their lives. If men experience problems in coming to terms with the termination, there is also the belief that they can solve it themselves and do not need to turn to others for help.

I saw something of this in myself. Celia wanted to get in touch with SATFA. I had no objection to that, but I was reluctant to get involved myself. I didn't think I needed to. I knew I had problems with coming to terms with the abnormality and our decision to have a termination, but I thought I could sort those out myself without anyone else's help, and perhaps like many men in this situation I wanted to put the experience behind me and get on with my life.

Why was I, and why are other men, reluctant to talk in these situations? I have no evidence to support my view but I believe it can arise from a number of things. The whole episode might be seen as the woman's problem; it was she who bore the child and had the termination. Soon afterwards men return to work and, although this will bring stress, the air of normality can crowd out the worries and emotions about the termination. Men may, therefore, appear unaffected and may not recognize their own needs.

My own experience was that whatever reluctance I felt about reliving the experience, once I started to talk it became easier. Although I did not realize it at the start, I found that I did need to talk about how I felt. Talking was painful; at times I just wanted to shut the memories away, but then I discovered that it could be a release. I became more honest with myself and articulated emotions that I had not always been fully aware of. Talking helped me to grieve, to understand my own actions and to find a place in my life for all that had happened.

The reluctance that many men feel about talking is also not helped by circumstances, because they do not often find themselves in situations with appropriate opportunities to talk about what has happened. Certainly you can talk about these things with your partner, but as I have already said, in circumstances where a father may find that he is having to adopt a supportive role, this may not be easy. Anyway, what may be needed, for both, is to talk to someone else. However, unless you are fortunate, a man is much less likely to find opportunities to talk than a woman. The kind of subject that might naturally lead to talk about a termination is much more likely to arise in discussion between women than between men.

Men also usually return to work shortly after the termination. That is not a place where the topic of a termination for abnormality will be likely to arise, or one which is likely to encourage talk of that kind. Even where there is goodwill, if you have to be tough and hard-nosed in your job it is difficult to unburden your inner feelings at the same time. This is not to say that employers are always lacking in compassion, but while at work demands are made of you and, after the initial expressions of sympathy, a prolonged problem or absence may itself become an issue. No matter how good your relationship with your colleagues it is a different one to the personal relationships you might have outside work. I talked to my colleagues and explained what had happened and what we had decided. It helped to talk, but at the same time I was not entirely sure that I wanted to go into all this with those I worked with. In an environment in which you are expected to perform, and are judged on that performance, people are wary of disclosing matters of this personal kind.

If I am right about male psychology and the lack of opportunities men have to talk, can anything be done to help? I believe that counselling would be of value but comment from fathers suggests that few are offered any professional counselling. I did not receive any counselling, but through SATFA I became involved with a self-help group which my wife was helping to organize. I had doubts about joining in but, despite those doubts and inhibitions, I found that it was beneficial. We had all been through the experience, and were there just to talk and listen. In that supportive atmosphere I found that I articulated emotions and feelings that I had not fully recognized before. Even listening to other people was helpful because not only did it enable me to recognize my own feelings, but meeting other people who had come to terms with their grief also helped me to see that it was possible to work through this tragedy.

Although I found enormous benefit from that self-help group it is not the answer for everyone, and such groups have their limitations. Women are in the majority in most meetings and this in itself will deter some men from talking or even attending. The composition of a group will also affect the atmosphere. On the few occasions I have been in an all male group there has been a difference in tone and topic. If nothing else, being away from your partner can give some extra freedom to talk.

A FINAL REFLECTION

Some 6 years have now passed since our termination and, although the pain has largely gone, one does not forget. As a parent I value the medical advances which enable the detection of fetal abnormality, but such developments have a cost. Ordinary and usually unsuspecting people are put in a position where they have to take a most difficult decision. I believe that parents should have that right, but it is important to remember that, while ending the life of an unborn baby may avoid one tragedy, it may, unless both parents are cared for, itself create another.

FURTHER READING

O'Dowd, T. (1993) The needs of fathers. *British Medical Journal*, **306**, 1484–1485

13

Looking in from the outside –

reactions to a termination of pregnancy for fetal abnormality from the point of view of those who care

Margaretha White-van Mourik

Judge no man before you have walked a mile in his moccasins
(Indian proverb; Arizona)

You cannot prevent the birds of sadness and sorrow from
circling above your head, but you can prevent them from
making nests in your hair (Chinese proverb)

INTRODUCTION

Couples who embark on a pregnancy expect to have a 'normal'
child, yet 2% will have an abnormal outcome. Until 20 years ago
there was no choice but to accept the risks distributed by nature.
If fate gave you a defective child you accepted it as well as you
could and then learned to live with the consequent and perpetual
grief. Parents who were aware of a genetic problem within their
family may have avoided having any children because their fear
of having an abnormal child outweighed their desire for offspring. They subsequently suffered the sadness of not realizing
their desired family.

Developments in obstetrics, biochemistry and cytology, con-
current with the introduction in Britain of laws which allow
abortion for fetal abnormality, have opened the road to antenatal

screening and prenatal diagnosis. These combined advances now provide couples with choice. Testing a baby before birth for genetic or other major abnormalities is a growing and rapidly changing field of medicine. But at the same time, these tests raise some agonizing ethical dilemmas: despite the scientific advances, intervention usually provides one choice; to terminate a pregnancy or not.

In this chapter we will examine what happens to couples when an 'act of God' transforms into an act of their own choosing, and what practical, ethical, spiritual, emotional and social issues are involved in trying to live with the decision to terminate a pregnancy for fetal abnormality. We will explore how as carers and as society as a whole we can reduce the emotional burden of this choice.

AN OUTSIDER'S CONFRONTATION WITH THE PSYCHOSOCIAL
CONSEQUENCES OF A TERMINATION OF PREGNANCY FOR
FETAL ABNORMALITY

In 1982 I was asked to recruit patients for the Medical Research Council Vitamin Study. This study was designed to discover whether recurrences of neural tube defects could be reduced by taking certain vitamins before conception. The majority of couples approached had experienced a termination of pregnancy for neural tube defect in the recent or distant past. Over the next 10 years I visited about 1200 of these couples at home and had the opportunity to stay in touch with many for the duration of the study. It was on these occasions that I learned about the intensity of grief felt by many, a grief that for some was as painful and vivid 5 years after the event as it had been at the time. I noticed that there were great differences in coping with the intervention and its aftermath but that there were certain emotions and difficulties that many had in common. I wondered at the time about the medical care, follow-up and support given to these couples and will refer to studies reporting on these issues. I observed the difficulties for carers too.

Many couples found it extremely difficult to ask for help or accept support after the intervention in spite of experiencing difficulties. Many found it easier to accept this support in the framework of a research programme but reflected years later on how helpful it had been and how much they had needed it.

In this chapter we will explore the reasons for these reactions and try to discover ways to overcome difficulties in providing care.

IDENTIFICATION WITH THE FETUS

Some sections of our society are still astonished by the grief reactions of couples after fetal loss. One of the reasons for this may be that western cultures have still not decided officially on the status of the human embryo (Reilly, 1979; Dunstan, 1988). Some other cultures have traditionally had personification of the fetus before birth (Cranley, 1981a). The relationship with the fetus starts after the awareness of pregnancy; thus the Siriona of East Bolivia perform the same bereavement ritual for a miscarried fetus as for a deceased adult. In Cambodia the dead fetus is believed to have magical protective powers and is honoured after birth (Walter, 1980).

Cranley (1981b), reporting on the relationship of parents with their 'unborn', noted that there was a wealth of interaction between the mother and her fetus. She observed that both father and mother developed bonding behaviour towards the fetus. She perceived that this phenomenon displayed an involvement with the fetus in which the fetus is experienced as a future child.

Although the infant–mother relationship develops gradually, quickening (maternal awareness of the fetal movements in the 14th–20th week of pregnancy) was often seen as a milestone (Bibring and Valenstein, 1967; Hollerbach, 1979). New developments in diagnostic techniques have been shown to induce an earlier and more intense involvement with the fetus (Reading *et al.*, 1981; Fletcher and Evans, 1983; Blumberg, 1984). Fetal life is now audible (fetal heart sounds) and visible (ultrasonography) from 8–10 weeks, and these techniques present the mother with undeniable evidence of fetal life (Lumley, 1980). It is not unusual for the first ultrasound picture to be saved as the first photograph of the child.

FETAL LOSS, GRIEF AND MOURNING

With parental awareness of the fetus as an independent identity, it is not surprising that the loss of a wanted and planned pregnancy is experienced as the loss of a child. Many women who abort spontaneously experience anguish, loneliness and depression following the realization of pregnancy loss (Pasnau and Farah, 1977; Borg and Lasker, 1982). Where there was ambivalence toward the pregnancy there could be guilt feelings. A sense of physical inadequacy and responsibility for the loss is shared by many.

The response to fetal loss is appropriately viewed as a form of bereavement (Lloyd and Laurence, 1985). Grieving is not a pathological symptom but a normal, and even necessary, reaction after fetal loss (Pedder, 1982). The duration of the reaction depends on the success with which the individual does 'grief work', which chiefly entails the acceptance of the feelings of intense distress. Avoiding these feelings and denying what has happened may lead to 'morbid grief', which is either a delayed reaction precipitated by specific circumstances or events, sometimes years later, or a distorted reaction which may be difficult to recognize as the original grief. This unresolved grief may in turn have an adverse affect on health (Stroebe and Stroebe, 1987).

It is often assumed that the longer the period of gestation, the closer the bonding to the fetus and therefore the greater the feelings of bereavement after pregnancy loss. However, just as not all births of live healthy babies result in immediate and ideal attachment, so women with first or second trimester pregnancy loss must not be assumed to have a less severe reaction to bereavement. More important criteria are:

- the significance of the pregnancy to the parents;
- their previous experience of loss and adaptation to it;
- their personalities;
- their perception of social support.

TERMINATION OF PREGNANCY FOR FETAL ABNORMALITY

Prenatal diagnosis is now available for many couples with a family history of genetic disease thus enabling them to dare to consider further pregnancies. Antenatal maternal serum screening for detection of neural tube defects and Down syndrome is offered to an increasing number of pregnant women. Cystic fibrosis screening is being explored in pilot studies. In these cases there is the option of terminating the pregnancy when an affected fetus is diagnosed. The emotional implications of screening and prenatal diagnosis are many and complex but I will concentrate on professional observation of the couples who were subjected to the acute trauma imparted by the discovery of fetal defect and who chose the option of termination of pregnancy.

The realization of an unfavourable result triggers an immediate grief response that may be characterized by disbelief, shock and anger (Blumberg, 1974; Donnai, Charles and Harris, 1981; Adler and Kusnick, 1982). Hopes and expectations are dashed by the revelation of the fetal abnormality. The medico-legal necessity of a quick decision (caused by the previous 28-week time limit for termination in Britain) either to continue or terminate the pregnancy adds to the burden of the already distressed couple. Previous abstract attitudes towards abortion appeared to provide little guidance for couples trapped in this moral dilemma. The parents understanding of the specific defect affecting the fetus is a significant determinant of their course of decision and action. (Blumberg, 1984; Korenromp *et al.*, 1992).

PSYCHOSOCIAL CONSEQUENCES

In contrast to the mostly positive reactions of women after an abortion for psychosocial indications (Doane and Quigley, 1981; Adler *et al.*, 1990), many authors (Lloyd and Laurence, 1985; Thomassen-Brepols, 1985; Black, 1989; Frets *et al.*, 1990; White-van Mourik, Connor and Ferguson-Smith, 1992; Korenromp *et al.*, 1992) have observed the opposite following a termination of pregnancy for fetal abnormality. When the findings in the literature are collated, the reasons for the increased distress emerge. The majority of women who agreed to antenatal screening or prenatal diagnosis had planned and/or welcomed the pregnancy. All were in the second trimester of their pregnancy and those who agreed to screening had often not seriously considered an abnormal result. The intervention thus had the psychological meaning of the loss of a wanted child. Loss implies mourning, yet coping and grieving were complicated by other problems which needed attention, such as the perceived loss of biological, moral and social competence and the associated loss of self-esteem. Conflicting emotions were subsequently complicated by two conflicting images: the image of the wished for, fantasized baby and the image of the damaged or handicapped child (Thomassen-Brepols, 1985).

ASPECTS OF COPING IN THE SHORT TERM

The first reaction reported by most couples immediately after the termination of pregnancy procedure was a feeling of relief that it was over. Many felt numbed by the diagnosis and the agonizing decisions that had been made in the previous few days. For some this numbness continued during their stay as an inpatient; others became painfully aware of their loss during their time in hospital. Because many women are cared for in postnatal wards this awareness was reinforced by hearing babies cry yet seeing their own empty cot. Especially painful were questions regarding the baby's well being from fellow patients and well-meaning auxiliary staff. Low self-esteem was reinforced by the attitude and ward policies of staff. One woman told me that she had spoken to a fellow patient who had had a stillbirth.

> Although we both left hospital with empty arms, she had had the opportunity to hold her baby, which had been presented to her dressed and washed in a little Moses basket. She had keepsakes and her baby would be buried. The name of the baby was put in a hospital memorial book. I was offered none of these memories and although I could see the baby after asking for it, the midwife held my baby as if it was something distasteful, a request to have my baby's name put in the memorial book was refused because I had had a termination of pregnancy and it was against hospital policy.

Low self-esteem was further reinforced for some on returning home. Studies reported that half of the couples were not contacted by any member of the primary care team (general practitioner, midwife, health visitor) nor were they invited to the surgery or visited at home; yet 60% of the women in studies experienced breast engorgement and lactation lasting more than 5 days (Lloyd and Laurence, 1985; White-van Mourik, Connor and Ferguson-Smith, 1990). One woman said: 'I felt that the medical profession had lost interest in me. The faulty fetus was terminated, so that was the end of the problem. But for me my problems were just starting.'

The realization of an unfavourable result triggered an immediate grief response and this was frequently characterized by disbelief, shock and anger. It was in this frame of mind that couples had to make decisions about their fetus. It is therefore not unusual for some newly bereaved parents to start to experience feelings of doubt shortly after the termination of pregnancy. In a recent study (White-van Mourik, Connor and Ferguson-Smith, 1992) half of the women admitted that they felt ambivalent about their decision. This was often linked to a lack of understanding of the fetal defect. There were fears that the medical professionals might have made a mistake and that they were disapproved of for the act of terminating the pregnancy. Mothers whose fetus's abnormality had been identified by maternal serum screening had frequently only a vague comprehension of the fetal condition for which they had been offered the intervention. Doubts were particularly common in very young women (16–20 years), those belonging to a lower socioeconomic group and those in whom the severity of the defect was uncertain. When the problem was identified by routine ultrasonography most women did not perceive the burden of choice as a consequence of having the investigation. This was in contrast to the 40% of women who were identified as being at risk through a maternal serum screening programme and who felt that they had not considered fully the implications of accepting the test. Doubts in these groups were significantly lessened if, at a post-termination consultation, time was taken to explain the condition of the fetus, the nature of the anomaly or illness and the likely prognosis. Even where there had been initial doubts, 2 years after the intervention the great majority of couples felt at peace with their decision (Thomassen-Brepols, 1985; White-van Mourik, 1992).

REPORTED EMOTIONAL AND SOMATIC REACTIONS IN THE FIRST 6 MONTHS

It is common for a feeling of deep sadness to be shared by both partners after the termination of pregnancy. Depression, anger, fear, guilt and failure were the other most frequently mentioned strong emotions. The anger was often a reaction to the feeling of helplessness for not having been able to protect their child from harm. The feeling of responsibility for this new life was mentioned by some men, but was expressed principally by women. Feelings of guilt could be focused on various aspects: towards the child, because a decision was made that it should not live, towards a previous child with a similar defect and towards one's partner. When expressing their feelings about fear, couples stressed the possibility of recurrence of the abnormality and the idea of having to repeat the whole decision-making process. Having to face the consequences of that choice was, and for some remained, terrifying.

Some women complained of prolonged numbness, panic spells and palpitations, but only men admitted to feeling withdrawn and being excluded (Korenromp *et al.*, 1992; White-van Mourik, 1992). One male partner typically explained: 'Of course it hurts and making such a decision was emotionally draining, but I can't see how talking about it helps. I want to be left alone.'

In our society, reproduction and reproductive failure are still frequently perceived as the woman's preserve. One husband explained:

> Everyone asked how my wife felt but nobody seemed to consider that I had feelings too. Even when things went wrong, the obstetrician explained all about it to my wife and her mother and by the time I came home from work (they did not want to worry me) they had more or less decided to terminate my baby. I felt so angry and redundant, but could not show it as my wife was upset and needed me.

As well as coping with strong feelings many couples report somatic symptoms. Of these, listlessness, loss of concentration, irritability and crying are mentioned most frequently. Male partners found that a lack of concentration in the first few months led to mistakes at work and to unexpected failures in exams.

Nightmares commonly have one or more of three elements:

- **replay**, in which the termination procedure is repeated night after night, and sometimes continues intermittently for up to a year after the termination of pregnancy;
- **persecution**, in which the parent runs away to prevent pursuers from taking the baby;
- **blame**, in which the baby, or family members, appears and accuses the parent of murder.

Despite these dissonant feelings and complaints, many couples felt reluctant to bring them up in discussion with health professionals, family or friends for fear of being judged mentally unstable or weak. This reticence may be overcome by carefully formulated questions asked as part of the routine post-termination protocol.

LONG-TERM PSYCHOSOCIAL AND COPING ASPECTS

Two years after the termination of pregnancy, most couples reported that they had regained their equilibrium. For some this happened less than 6 months after the intervention. However, most continued to experience sadness about the loss of the baby and to fear recurrence of the condition in a subsequent pregnancy. The feeling of continuing relief was especially mentioned by those families familiar with a distressing handicap or genetic disease.

In two studies (Thomassen-Brepols, 1985; White-van Mourik, 1992), about 20% of women continued to feel angry, guilty, a failure, irritable and tearful. They felt that these strong emotions had a disruptive impact on their lives and relationships. Men appeared to come to terms with their loss more quickly than their spouses. The same analysis was made by Martinson *et al.* (1980) who observed that after the loss of a child, fathers were twice as likely as mothers to report that the most intensive part of grieving was over in a few weeks. However, their response may have reflected the social expectations of the father 'to take it like a man'. Men appear to have a greater need to keep their grief private (De Frain, Taylor and Ernst, 1982) and this may even give their partners the impression that they are not affected by the loss, yet it was often the male partners who were more apprehensive about the idea of a further pregnancy.

THE MARITAL RELATIONSHIP

Many partners reported an initial closeness after the termination of pregnancy. They found that the procedure and the deep emotions after the intervention had brought a new dimension to the relationship. Where there had been a close relationship before the intervention, partners generally were able to be understanding and supportive. Where difficulties were experienced, these were reported to be most pronounced after 3–6 months and appeared to be due to lack of communication, irritation and an intolerance of the different coping mechanisms used in coming to terms with the bereavement. Severe difficulties appeared where there were unspoken attributions of guilt and blame between the partners.

Sexual problems arose where the partners experienced

different needs and were unable to communicate them. The woman might have difficulties separating the sexual act from pregnancy and conception, while the man might want to reinforce emotional closeness, or vice versa. In a few cases, sexual difficulties had continued over many years post-termination without help being sought (White-van Mourik, 1992).

THE OTHER CHILDREN IN THE FAMILY

About half the couples noticed a change in their behaviour towards their other children. The majority treasured them more but felt overprotective and allowed them less freedom. The realization that it was possible for bad luck to strike twice was strong. For some the feeling of overprotectiveness became a worry and they had difficulties coping with their anxiety. About 20% of the women interviewed were so preoccupied with their grief that their children were a source of irritation for them. In rare cases there was a feeling of total indifference towards the other children in the family and some children were cared for by other relatives for weeks or months. When the women felt negative about their children, they felt extremely guilty and never brought up the subject without being asked about it, yet discussing this guilt was reported to be a great relief.

FRIENDS AND FAMILY

In times of stress and uncertainty, the majority of people turn to their close friends and relatives for support. The majority of couples looked for different aspects of support in different relationships. Understanding, consideration and warm contact were hoped for in the relationship with their close family. Good listening, understanding and thoughtfulness were felt to be the most valued aspects of support from friends and to a lesser degree from colleagues and neighbours.

Couples expressed the need to feel that others were sensitive to their anguish and shared their feeling of loss. It was the relationships that meant the most to the couple which produced most friction: friends and relatives are often unsure how to help. In other situations the grieving couple may indicate what help is needed, but in the case of a termination for fetal abnormality they too are bewildered. Couples report conflicting feelings: of feeling grateful and angry, supported and isolated, rationally recognizing the prevention of the birth of a handicapped child and emotionally mourning the wanted baby. These conflicts were instrumental in the reluctance to instigate discussion which was evident in many couples.

Many people prefer to avoid the subjects of genetic inheritance, handicap and abortion, especially when they come 'too close to home'. This means that couples who already find it difficult to talk about their intervention are actively discouraged from doing so. When expressing grief and loss they were sometimes reminded by supporters that they had been lucky to have had the choice. This further created feelings of guilt and failure. Other supporters kept a well-intentioned silence that was readily misinterpreted as disapproval. It was frequently assumed by outsiders that a strong grief reaction was linked to regretting the termination, and silence was employed to prevent guilt in the couple. However, follow up after 2 years showed that most grieved but on reflection few regretted the termination (White-van Mourik, 1992). As time passed, women found it painful when those around them seemed totally unaware of the expected date of delivery and the anniversary of the termination.

MORAL DILEMMAS

Grieving after a termination for fetal abnormality is complicated by a loss of moral self-esteem, because there is an awareness of personal contribution to the pregnancy loss. Unlike miscarriage or stillbirth, the loss was not unavoidable but had been chosen. There is a confrontation with one's own morality in making decisions about life and death. Even the knowledge that the fetus would have died anyway does not take away the overwhelming sense of responsibility for this new life. The decision to terminate the pregnancy frequently conflicted with previously held beliefs about right and wrong. I interviewed women who had been staunch 'Pro-Lifers' who, before the intervention, could not have imagined being able to make a decision to terminate a pregnancy. This ethical conflict, and the moral pain of having to choose against life or for possible suffering, was strongly illustrated by the fact that many couples were searching for purpose or reason. Even those who normally did not have strong religious convictions reported preoccupation with a higher being; either to be angry with or to plead care for the child that they had not been able to protect. As a carer I found this deep anguish and continuing care for the lost child extremely moving, but I felt it difficult to give the right expression of support for this spiritual disturbance. Very few women got in touch with a religious leader (Thomassen-Brepols, 1985; White-van Mourik, 1992).

SUPPORT FROM THE MEDICAL COMMUNITY

Although hospital staff were reported to be kind and caring (White-van Mourik, 1990), few hospitals appeared to have a protocol concerning the discharge and follow-up procedures after the termination of pregnancy. This meant that it was not uncommon for the woman to turn up in the surgery of her family doctor only to be asked how the pregnancy was progressing. This was extremely painful for the bereaved women and embarrassing for their general practitioners who had not been informed. Even where there was kindness, ambivalence towards the termination of pregnancy was shown in subtle ways. Some hospitals, for instance, refused parents access to a memorial book. This book is kept to acknowledge babies lost after late miscarriage, stillbirth or neonatal death. Hospitals were unable to give convincing explanations for this.

There is reluctance in both men and women to report emotional disturbances or somatic complaints to the family doctor for fear of being put on tranquillizers or antidepressants or even being admitted to a psychiatric hospital. Empathy, good listening and an understanding of the subjective qualities of the experience were highly appreciated by the couple when given by members of the primary and obstetric care team. Equally important was clear, factual information about preconception care and recurrence risk for future pregnancies.

CONSIDERING FURTHER PREGNANCIES

Loss of biological self-esteem is one of the factors which affects couples after a termination for fetal abnormality. As with fetal loss, the birth of a handicapped child is still, if at times subconsciously, perceived to be reproductive failure. Feelings of shame and failure were frequently reinforced by the family and inlaws who would fervently declare that this abnormality could not come from their side of the family. This exaggerated the bereaved parents' loss of self-value, yet as observed in the literature about grief response (Thomassen-Brepols, 1985), a feeling of self esteem is an important ingredient in the coping strategy. Complicating the issue further is the increased incidence of fetal abnormality in subsequent pregnancies.

Most couples have a planned family size but the wish for more children may be amended by circumstances. In the past, couples at risk of genetic disease were often deterred from planning further pregnancies (Emery, Watt and Clark, 1972, 1973; Reynolds, Puck and Robinson, 1974; Klein and Wyss, 1977). Many authors reported changed reproductive behaviour after the introduction of prenatal diagnosis in that couples dared to try to achieve their planned family (Modell *et al.*, 1984; Kaback *et al.*, 1984; Scriver *et al.*, 1984; Modell and Bulyzhenkov, 1988; Evers-Kiebooms *et al.*, 1988). The decision-making process was perceived to be more burdensome by the couples who decided to have children using the option of prenatal diagnosis than it was by those for whom prenatal diagnosis was not available (Frets *et al.*, 1990). The literature about the sequelae of a termination for fetal abnormality provides anecdotal information about couples refraining from further pregnancy. Only two studies examined the reproductive behaviour of couples after a termination for fetal abnormality (Thomassen-Brepols, 1985, De Frain, Taylor and Ernst, 1982). In the Thomassen-Brepols study, where 40% of the women were 38 years and over, half the women experienced a reproductive conflict. In another study, (White-van Mourik, 1989) the mean maternal age was 27 years and only 6% of the women were over 38 years of age. Perhaps for this reason only 14% experienced a reproductive conflict. The women in conflict were torn between their desire for another child and their fear of recurrence of the abnormality and the subsequent decision process.

These two studies confirmed Lippmann-Hands and Fraser's view (1979) that neither the objective interpretation of the recurrence risk nor single factors such as religious conviction, negative feeling about the termination procedure or lack of support post-termination necessarily deterred couples from further reproduction. The deciding factors in the reproductive conflict after a termination for fetal abnormality are:

- maternal age;
- an unexpected diagnosis;
- the presence of children in the family;
- a subtle combination of factors.

Frets *et al.* (1990) made a similar observation in genetic counsellees.

The reason that the risk of procreational conflict is largest among older women is that for them time is running out, with the end of fertility approaching. Not only did this group have to contend with the losses described in the sequelae of termination for abnormality, they frequently experienced disapproval for their desire for further pregnancies from their spouse, relatives and friends, especially if they had other children. Another group who wanted more children but often decided against further pregnancies were women who had received an unexpected diagnosis, i.e. one different from the one for which they may have requested prenatal diagnosis (Leschot, Verjaal and Treffers, 1982; Thomassen-Brepols, 1985). Previous knowledge of fetal abnormality was helpful not only during the decision-making process, but also in attempts to come to terms with the termination of pregnancy; thus a surprise diagnosis reinforced the perceived loss of biological competence and decreased the feeling of self-value. Help could be offered to couples with such a conflict by providing focused counselling. In this the counsellor focuses on the counsellee's feelings concerning the reproductive decision, accepts apparently irrational considerations (because these feelings indicate the influence of unconscious motives) and understands the role which guilt plays in the decision (Frets *et al.*, 1990).

All women who subsequently became pregnant in the Thomassen-Brepols (1985) and White-van Mourik (1989) studies chose prenatal diagnosis.

THE NEW BABY

The birth of a new baby was frequently the climax to a worrying time and most parents were totally delighted with their healthy child. Unfortunately this delight was often coloured with sadness by the memory of the last delivery. A few women admitted to having a pregnancy too soon after their loss in order to try to alleviate the pain of their grief. The birth of a healthy child may in these cases start a renewed grieving pattern. One woman said:

> When he was put in my arms I suddenly realized what I had missed last time, and the only thing I could do was cry. I must have cried for weeks and felt so ungrateful for feeling so intensely sad. My husband and parents were totally bewildered, because I had been so good after the termination of pregnancy.

Understanding of these feelings by those carers attending the postnatal parents was found to be extremely helpful.

LIVING WITH THE CHOICE

The issue brought up most frequently after the termination was that of confusion concerning the ethical status of the decision. Directions may have been given regarding tests, the condition of the fetus, the admission to hospital and the termination procedure. This may not have been done very well but at least there was a system. However, when the termination was completed all became vague. Medical and social responsibility frequently seemed to have come to an end. The choices had been offered and the couples themselves had made the decisions. As has been discussed, for many couples and especially for those unfamiliar with the diagnosed fetal abnormality, the long process of realization, grieving and resolution was just starting. Unfortunately, few hospitals have a protocol for aftercare or long-term follow-up. Few couples are given the information about the psychosocial sequelae of the intervention or are helped to explore the coping strategies for coming to terms with the decision. Barbara Katz Rothman (1986) observed that:

> These women are victims of a social system that fails to take collective responsibility for the needs of its members, and leaves individual women to make impossible choices. We are spared collective responsibility, because we individualize the problem. We make it the woman's own. She chooses, and so we owe her nothing. Whatever the cost, she has chosen. It is her problem not ours.

In view of this, surely it should be an integral part of all antenatal screening programmes and diagnostic services not only to provide choice but to help couples to learn to live with this choice?

Many times in the past new directions in screening and prenatal diagnosis have been funded for their scientific development while neglecting funding for research into the psychosocial consequences of them.

CARE PROGRAMMES

No care, however thoughtful and thorough, can take away the pain of loss; neither can reassuring remarks take away moral anguish. Resolution of grief does not mean forgetting the event, as many women who lost babies decades ago could testify. Support can be provided by recognizing that the turmoil of feelings after a termination of pregnancy may be disabling but is not usually pathological and by helping couples who have difficulties unravelling their ambivalence.

This was confirmed in the perinatal mortality programmes which started to gain popularity in the mid-1980s (Bourne and Lewis, 1984; Kirk, 1984; Kellner, Donnelly and Gould, 1984). These programmes were instigated to gain greater awareness of psychological problems of families after a stillbirth or neonatal death. They allowed, and then encouraged, bereavement processes to run their course until a resolution of grief occurred. An immediate pregnancy to counteract the grieving process was discouraged. Forrest *et al.* (1982) mentioned that the duration of bereavement reactions was appreciably shortened by support and counselling. An important strategy was to encourage parents to hold and see their dead baby so that farewells could be said and thus provide an end to a process that started with the discovery and confirmation of the pregnancy. The reality of the farewell facilitated the grieving process that made resolution possible. In another study (White-van Mourik, 1989), the women who most deeply regretted not seeing their fetus were those who were too frightened or too tired to request a viewing after the termination of pregnancy procedure. They would have welcomed a picture of the fetus on file. It is indeed not uncommon for women to ring the hospital a decade after the intervention to request a picture of the fetus.

Self-help groups have been seen as invaluable in supporting women by reducing isolation (Vachon *et al.*, 1980). Their role in public relations and their help in the education of professionals has done much to raise public awareness of the problems.

COUPLES' PERCEPTION OF GOOD MANAGEMENT

When couples were asked for their recommendations on good management, three themes clearly emerged: recognition, information and hope (White-van Mourik, 1992).

Recognition

Recognition was described in several ways:

- as the confirmation of the couple's status as parents by medical staff, relatives and friends;
- as perception and comprehension of the grief;
- as an insight into the fact that apparent choice is often perceived as no choice at all but as the only action feasible under the circumstances for the couple;
- as an understanding of the fear of social disapproval and the subsequent reticence to ask for help when required;
- as perception of the turmoil of ambivalent feelings and the time it may take to come to terms with the event.

Recognition helps to boost the couple's self-esteem by making them feel normal under the circumstances. It prevents trivialization and the use of platitudes.

Information

Information and communication were found to be of enormous value in coming to terms with the termination of pregnancy for fetal abnormality. Explanations using appropriate language about the fetal abnormality, the termination of pregnancy procedure and preparation for the physical, psychosocial, short- and long-term sequelae were considered essential. An exploration of how to cope with feelings of anger, depression and irritability was appreciated. Better and continuing communication minimized the feeling of being out of control and reduced misunderstanding.

Hope

Hope for another pregnancy was felt to be of great importance to those wishing to achieve their planned family. A successful subsequent pregnancy counterbalanced the loss of biological self-esteem and to some extent restored a sense of social competence. Couples attached great importance to discussions about the implications of the fetal abnormality for further pregnancies, prenatal diagnosis and preconception health care.

PRACTICAL CONSIDERATIONS FOR THOSE WHO CARE

All couples should be given information about possible sequelae. They need an assessment of their coping strategies and encouragement to take steps to counteract their lack of self-esteem, but not all couples need long-term counselling. Within the context of continuing medical care, professionals have a responsibility to understand this new kind of grief and to recognize the signs that may indicate a need for further counselling or professional mental health intervention. Some groups may have particular problems in expressing their anxieties. Most men find it hard to 'open up' for fear of showing emotions and tears. It is therefore important to see the couple together. Those without a support network and those with a vulnerable personality prior to the termination need extra care. Those who had not coped with an antecedent bereavement experience have an increased risk of a poor outcome. For young, immature couples (between 16 and 20 years), it is often particularly hard to come to terms with the termination. Their moral convictions are frequently more 'black and white', their self-esteem is often lower and their peers have less experience or interest in bereavement processes. In addition they are frequently patronized by parents and medical professionals and are more timid about expressing themselves. Others who may need more time are couples who have communication difficulties and those with a reproductive conflict after the termination for fetal abnormality

Carers must ensure that they have channels to unload themselves as the intense pain and distress experienced by many couples can, at times, have a cumulative effect on one's own outlook on life.

Finally, regional audit of communication, provision of information and criteria of service will ensure that standards are being upheld.

REFERENCES

Adler, N.E., Henry, P.D., Major, B.N. *et al.* (1990) Psychological responses after abortion. *Science,* **248**, 41–44.

Adler, B. and Kusnick, T. (1982) Genetic counselling in prenatally diagnosed trisomy 18 and 21. *Paediatrics,* **69**, 94–99.

Bibring, B.L and Valenstein, A.F. (1967) The psychological aspects of pregnancy. *Clinical Obstetrics and Gynecology,* **19**, 357–371.

Black, R.B. (1989) A 1 and 6 month follow-up of prenatal diagnosis patients who lost pregnancies. *Prenatal Diagnosis,* **9**, 795–804.

Blumberg, B.D. (1974) Psychic sequelae of selective abortion. Yale University MD thesis.

Blumberg, B.D. (1984) The emotional implications of prenatal diagnosis, in *Psychological Aspects of Genetic Counselling,* (eds A.E.H. Emery and I.M. Pullen), Academic Press, London, pp. 202–217.

Borg, S. and Lasker, J. (1982) *When Pregnancy Fails: Coping with Miscarriage, Stillbirth and Infant Death,* Routledge & Kegan Paul, London.

Bourne, S. and Lewis, E. (1984) Delayed psychological effects of perinatal deaths: the next pregnancy and the next generation. *British Medical Journal,* **289**, 147–188.

Cranley, M.S. (1981a) Roots of attachment: the relationship of parents with their unborn, in *Perinatal Parental Behaviour: Nursing Research and Implications for the Newborn Health,* (eds R.P. Lederman, B.S. Raff and P. Caroll), Alan R. Liss, New York, pp. 59–83.

Cranley, M.S. (1981b) Development of a tool for measurement of maternal attachment during pregnancy. *Nurse Research,* **30**, 281–284.

De Frain, J., Taylor, J. and Ernst, L. (1982) *Coping with Sudden Infant Death,* Lexington Books, D.C. Heath, Lexington, MA.

Doane, B.K. and Quigley, B.G. (1981) Psychiatric aspects of therapeutic abortion (review article). *Canadian Medical Association Journal,* **125**, 427–432.

Donnai, P., Charles, N. and Harris, R. (1981) Attitudes of patients after genetic termination of pregnancy. *British Medical Journal,* **282**, 621–622.

Dunstan, G.R. (1988) Screening for fetal and genetic abnormality: social and ethical issues. *Journal of Medical Genetics,* **25**, 290–293.

Emery, A.E.H., Watt, M.S. and Clark, E.R. (1972) The effects of genetic counselling in Duchenne muscular dystrophy. *Clinical Genetics,* **3**, 147–150.

Emery, A.E.H., Watt, M.S. and Clark, E.R. (1973) Social effects of genetic counselling. *British Medical Journal,* **1**, 724–726.

Evers-Kiebooms, G., Denayer, L., Cassiman, J.J. and van den Berghe, H. (1988) Family planning decisions after the birth of a cystic fibrosis child: impact of prenatal diagnosis. *Scandanavian Journal of Gastroenterology,* **143**(suppl), 38–46.

Fletcher, J.C. and Evans, M.I. (1983) Maternal bonding in early fetal ultrasound examinations. *New England Journal of Medicine,* **308**, 392–393.

Forrest, G.C., Standish, E. and Baum, J.D. (1982) Support after perinatal death: a study of support and counselling perinatal bereavement. *British Medical Journal*, **285**, 1475–1479.

Frets, P.G., Los, F.J., Sachs, E.S. and Jahoda, M.G.J. (1990) Psychological counselling of couples experiencing a pregnancy termination after amniocentesis. *Journal of Psychosomatic Obstetrics and Gynecology*, **11**(special issue 1), 53–59.

Hollerbach, P.E. (1979) Reproductive attitudes and the genetic counsellee, in *Counselling in Genetics*, (eds Y.E. Hsia, K. Hirschorn, R.L. Silverberg and L. Godmillow), Alan R. Liss, New York, pp. 155–222.

Kaback, M., Zippin, D., Boyd, P. *et al.* (1984) Attitudes towards prenatal diagnosis of cystic fibrosis amongst parents of affected children, in *Cystic Fibrosis: Horizons*, (ed. D. Lawson), John Wiley, New York, pp. 6–28.

Kellner, K.R., Donnelly, W.H. and Gould, S.D. (1984) Parental behaviour after perinatal death: lack of predictive demography and obstetric variables. *Obstetrics and Gynecology* **63**, 809–814.

Kirk, E.P. (1984) Psychological effects and management of perinatal loss. *American Journal of Obstetrics and Gynecology*, **149**, 46–51.

Klein, D. and Wyss, D. (1977) Retrospective and follow-up study of approximately 1000 genetic consultations. *Journal of Human Genetics*, **25**, 47–57.

Korenromp, M.J., Iedema-Kuiper. H.R., van Spijker, H.G. *et al.* (1992) Termination of pregnancy on genetic grounds: coping with grieving. *Journal of Psychosomatic Obstetrics and Gynaecology*, **13**, 93–105.

Leschot, N.J., Verjaal, M. and Treffers, P.E. (1982) Therapeutic abortion on genetic indication; a detailed follow-up study of 20 patients. *Journal of Psychosomatic Obstetrics and Gynaecology*, **1**, 47–56.

Lippman-Hands, A. and Fraser, F.C. (1979) Genetic counselling: the provision and perception of information. *American Journal of Medical Genetics*, **3**, 113–127

Lloyd, J. and Laurence, K.M. (1985) Sequelae and support after termination of pregnancy for fetal malformation. *British Medical Journal*, **290**, 907–909.

Lumley J. (1980) The image of the fetus in the first trimester. *Birth and Family*, **7**, 5–14.

Martinson, I., Modow, D. and Henry, W. (1980) *Home Care for the Child with Cancer. Final Report.* (Grant no. Ca 19490). National Cancer Institute, US Department of Health and Human Services, Washington, DC.

Modell, B. and Bulyzhenkov, V. (1988) Distribution and control of some genetic disorders. *World Health Statistics Quarterly*, **41**, 209–218.

Modell, B., Petrou M., Ward R.H. *et al.* (1984) Effect of fetal diagnostic testing on birthrate of thalassaemia major in Britain. *Lancet*, **ii**, 1383–1386.

Pasnau, R. and Farah, J. (1977) Loss and mourning after abortion, in *The Family in Mourning*, (eds C. Hollingworth and R. Pasnau), Grune & Stratton, New York.

Pedder, J.R. (1982) Failure to mourn, and melancholia. *British Journal of Psychiatry*, **141**, 329–337.

Reading, A., Sledgemere, C.M., Campbell, S. *et al.* (1981) Psychological effects on the mother, of real-time ultrasound in antenatal clinics. *British Journal of Radiology*, **54**, 546.

Reilly, P. (1979) Genetic counselling: a legal perspective, in *Counselling in Genetics*, (eds Y.E. Hsia, K. Hirschorn, R.L. Silverberg and L. Godmillow), Alan R. Liss, New York, pp. 311–328

Reynolds, B.D., Puck, M.H. and Robinson, A. (1974) Genetic counselling: an appraisal. *Clinical Genetics*, **5**, 177–178.

Rothman, B.K. (1986) *The Tentative Pregnancy: Prenatal Diagnosis and the Future of Motherhood*, Viking Penguin, New York.

Scriver, C.R., Bardanis, M., Cartier, L. *et al.* (1984) Beta-thalassemia disease prevention; genetic medicine applied. *American Journal of Human Genetics*, **36**, 1024–1038.

Stroebe, W. and Stroebe, M. (1987) *Bereavement and Health, the Psychological and Physical Consequences of Partner Loss*, Cambridge University Press, Cambridge, pp. 168–223.

Thomassen-Brepols, L.J. (1985) Psychosociale aspecten van prenatale diagnostiek (Psychosocial aspects of prenatal diagnosis). Erasmus Universiteit, Rotterdam, PhD thesis.

Vachon, M.L.S., Lyall, W.A.L., Rogers, J. *et al.* (1980) A controlled study of self-help intervention for widows. *American Journal of Psychiatry*, **137**, 380–384.

Walter, C. (1980) The mipa: a social belief of peasants. *Revisita Latinoamericana de Psicologia*, **12**, 293–312

White-van Mourik M.C.A. (1989) The psycho-social sequelae of a termination of pregnancy for fetal abnormality. MSc Thesis. Glasgow: The University of Glasgow.

White-van Mourik, M.C.A., Connor, J.M. and Ferguson-Smith, M.A. (1990) Patient care before and after termination of pregnancy for neural tube defect. *Prenatal Diagnosis*, **10**, 497–505

White-van Mourik, M.C.A., Connor, J.M. and Ferguson-Smith, M.A. (1992) The psychosocial sequelae of a second-trimester termination of pregnancy for fetal abnormality. *Prenatal Diagnosis*, **12**, 189–204.

14

Caring for the carers

Elizabeth Friedrich

INTRODUCTION

The preceding chapters of this book have raised many issues and, while there are some answers, there are many more questions.

Staff in the health service are accustomed to dealing with dilemmas about appropriate treatment, about the patient's best interests, the patient's right to know. In the realm of obstetrics and paediatrics this is further complicated by the fact that there are two or more 'patients': the mother/parents and an actual or potential child. Nowhere are these issues more complex than in the area of prenatal diagnosis. Parents are often faced with what feel like impossible dilemmas and so, in their turn, are staff.

The issues that face staff are sometimes legal, sometimes moral and often simply existential ones of life, death, hope and disappointment. Often there are no answers. There is just supporting parents in difficult decisions (sometimes having to make those decisions), helping parents come to terms with loss and disappointment and supporting them through messy and untidy feelings. And then staff have to deal with their own feelings.

If health professionals are doing their best to care for patients in this situation, who is caring for the carer? Some health professionals may not even feel that this is an appropriate question. They may see no need to be cared for: it is not part of the medical model. Health professionals simply get on with the job, immune to the distress that might be caused to lesser mortals through all this contact with despair and death.

Is this true? Exposure to death, disease and distress has, to a certain extent, a desensitizing effect: staff learn to normalize them. But for most people there are still elements of their job that are shocking, distressing or just difficult. Health professionals are not immune to the depression, anxiety and other forms of mental illness that afflict 25% of the workforce at any one time (Jenkins, 1992). Health professionals have some of the highest occupational stress ratings (Cooper, Cooper and Eaker, 1988). Nurses are a much studied group who have been shown to have higher than average levels of smoking, alcohol consumption, absence rates and suicide (Hingley and Cooper, 1986).

Obstetricians, paediatricians and especially midwives have chosen to work in an area which in the main is associated with creation, new life, hope. At the cutting edge of developments in genetics the work is often associated with the loss of hope, the ending of life through termination of a pregnancy. This is distressing to parents and staff alike, and the sheer repetition of it can weigh heavily on staff.

STAFF SUPPORT

In October 1992 the National Association for Staff Support for staff in the health services (NASS) published *A Charter for Staff Support* (National Association for Staff Support, 1992). The opening paragraph states: 'Personal health care is often stressful and over a period of time staff may become worn out or burnt out. Staff support helps those who care for others to be fully effective in their service.'

The charter goes on to suggest that the damage to individuals and to the organization (in terms of absenteeism, turnover and poor work performance) can be largely prevented by:

- recognizing that stress exists;
- acknowledging the need for support;
- educating staff in the prevention and management of stress;
- providing adequate support services;
- creating a caring culture in the workplace;
- promoting good staff support practices throughout the system.

Before looking at the role of staff support in the context of workers in prenatal diagnosis and considering what can be done to identify and acknowledge the pressures and attendant stress, it is important to examine in a more general context the nature of stress.

STRESS

Stress is sometimes dismissed as a fashionable ailment which does not really exist. The physical and psychological symptoms of stress result from overstimulation of the fight/flight response, the complex physiological and biochemical reaction which takes place in our bodies when we are confronted with a situation we perceive as threatening or challenging. This process, which releases energy into the blood stream, increases our heart rate, quickens our breathing, tenses muscles and sharpens reflexes while slowing the process of digestion, can be life-saving when we are confronted with a physical challenge. When our response is physical our body is likely to return to its normal state fairly quickly. If the perceived threat is the pressure of work, anxiety about confronting a difficult patient or feeling inadequate in a demanding situation, there is no physical release from the situation and it may well be prolonged. The cumulative effect of frequent arousal combined with our tendency to want to deny or hide its effects can lead us to become stressed.

The useful short-term physical effects of arousal can, if repeated constantly, translate over time into breathing problems, chest pains, hypertension, muscle tension (especially in the back, shoulders and neck), digestive problems, irritable bowel, headaches, sexual and fertility problems, greater susceptibility to infection and a host of other problems (Cooper, Cooper and Eaker, 1988).

Instead of feeling alert, we begin to experience difficulty in concentrating and making decisions. We exhibit irritability, forgetfulness, lack of confidence, become hypercritical of ourselves and others, experience depression, anxiety, even panic attacks. So the more stressed we are, the less likely we are to be able to think rationally about ourselves and our situation. We are often unaware of our level of stress until someone else points it out to us.

Under stress our behaviour may change in a variety of ways. We may overeat, or experience loss of appetite, drink in excess, smoke more, or consume an excess of caffeine. We may have problems sleeping, become hyperactive, become more prone to accidents or withdraw socially and from our family.

No-one experiences all these symptoms, but in order to care for ourselves and minimize stress we have first to recognize not only that it exists but also the way in which it affects each of us personally, learning to identify our own symptoms and those of colleagues and staff for whom we are responsible. Having identified the symptoms, we need to recognize situations that trigger stress in us in order to try to avoid or change them. We also need to develop forms of relaxation to minimize the effects of stress.

Stress may be usefully defined as pressure that becomes unmanageable. An optimum amount of pressure is necessary for us to perform at our best – too little is as stressful as too much, as Figure 14.1 shows.

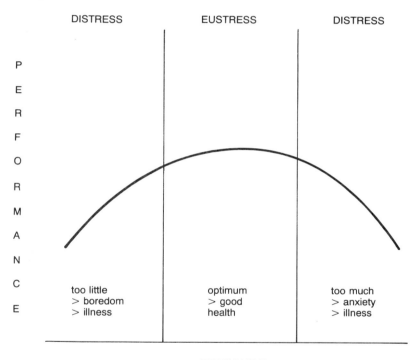

Figure 14.1 The relationship between pressure and performance (adapted from Cooper, Cooper and Eaker, 1988).

Eustress is the amount of pressure that produces the optimum performance and quality of life for any given individual.

Each individual has his or her own tolerance of pressure: what is exciting and stimulating for one will feel like an intolerable pressure for another. We may change our stress levels by reviewing some of the beliefs on which we operate, for example: 'I must be perfect', 'Only the best is good enough', 'I am always responsible', etc. However, our tolerance of pressure depends on our individual psychological make-up, our history, our education and training, our life experience and expectations.

STRESS CONNECTED WITH WORK IN PRENATAL DIAGNOSIS

To reduce stress we need to identify situations which we find stressful and to consider to what extent we can change them. Anyone working in the area of prenatal diagnosis will have to confront issues concerned with termination. Many of these are posed as questions to which we may feel we have no answers. Whose quality of life do we put first – that of the mother or that of the fetus? What degree of abnormality makes termination appropriate – and who should decide, parents, doctors, society? If we can offer tests for abnormalities, should we automatically do so? Is it right to terminate a pregnancy on the basis of the sex of the baby because it may carry a defective gene?

Anyone with strong views about this kind of issue who believes that there are absolute moral answers will be under considerable pressure if working with colleagues or patients who do not share these views. It may seem very obvious to suggest that someone who has these kind of difficulties should not be working in the field of prenatal diagnosis. Our career choices, however, are not always clear-cut. We may drift into a particular area of work without investigating every aspect of it. We change; the nature of the work changes. The choices presented to parents even 20 years ago were vastly different from those of today.

Someone who embarked on a midwifery career 20 years ago because she enjoyed delivering babies might rarely have encountered terminations. Today she might be asked to assist at a termination of a fetus that might be suffering from an inherited disorder or might turn out to be perfectly healthy. If an individual is unhappy in such a situation he or she needs to feel it is possible either to opt out of certain situations or perhaps to move to a different area of work. This can be difficult and takes courage. The organization and the department unit manager must be sensitive to the needs of such individuals.

Staff who are comfortable in a role advising and supporting parents in whatever choices they make still find themselves confronting painful situations. Terminating a pregnancy, even when it seems the only choice, is still a distressing experience. Late terminations, where a baby may be delivered alive, are particularly difficult for parents and staff. It can be just as distressing to watch on ultrasound as a fetus responds to a lethal injection.

Frequent involvement with terminations can lead to stress, and it is important not only that staff have support but that they are also given the opportunity to work in other areas as a reminder that pregnancy and birth can be a normal, uncomplicated event.

DEALING WITH STRESS

While there is an increasing recognition of occupational stress, there are still traditionalists who view it as namby-pamby or special pleading to admit a situation is stressful, feeling it would be unprofessional and tantamount to saying that they could not cope. Working in this kind of ethos it is difficult to say: 'I find this situation really difficult and distressing and I would like some help and support. In asking for this I am not being weak or inadequate, I am acting professionally and maturely.' But it is taking this kind of risk that will gradually begin to change the culture.

It is the same fear of seeming unable to cope that can prevent staff from drawing on the support of one another. Much stress can be relieved by simply talking things through with a colleague, acknowledging a painful decision, the anxiety that it might not lead to a satisfactory outcome, just having someone else say 'how awful; what a lousy situation'. Of course many staff do use one another in this way. Giving staff permission to acknowledge stress needs to apply at every level: not just doctors saying it is difficult for nurses, midwives or ultrasonographers but owning up to their own stress, the difficulty of not having answers. This of course goes against the hierarchical nature of the health service.

When a group of staff are involved in an event, or a series of events that they find particularly distressing, they may need more than informal support from one another. Work with people involved in traumatic events suggests that the degree to which people suffer post traumatic symptoms (anxiety, reliving the event, sleeping difficulties, withdrawing socially, panic attacks) can be reduced by providing debriefing after the event (Wright, 1989). Staff are brought together to discuss the event in a non-judgemental setting. Each member of staff is invited to describe their experience. This soon reveals that the degree to which an individual is affected does not necessarily relate to the degree of their involvement in the event. The staff group as a whole will often experience a degree of catharsis, and individual's experiences can be heard and acknowledged. Handled sympathetically, this kind of discussion will help improve staff morale.

There will be times when an event at work or at home, or often a combination of the two, will trigger in an individual overwhelming feelings of anxiety and stress. Support from other staff members or a manager may not be enough. In these circumstances the member of staff is often referred to the occupational health department. It is useful if the manager also knows of an accessible counselling service, whether in-house or available locally. Staff who are not comfortable with the idea of seeking counselling and go under duress will not benefit from it, but often staff have mistaken ideas about counselling, associating it with mental illness or notions of failure. An explanation that the aim of counselling is to help them rediscover their own resources and the provision of information about access to a service can encourage a staff member to seek help before a problem becomes a crisis.

Stress can often be prevented by teamwork and better planning of patient care. It need not happen that a patient is told different things by different professionals, or that one professional does not know what another has said. The dilemmas discussed in Chapter 7 are sometimes unavoidable but often not. It may be a matter of designing consultations around the patient's needs instead of those of the organization, of being clear where responsibility lies for giving information and of providing the appropriate time and privacy for counselling a patient and providing appropriate training for staff at all levels. This may have time implications as well as financial ones. However, not feeling rushed and being dealt with sympathetically are what patients want, as is evident from the patients quoted in earlier chapters. Meeting the needs of patients has the added bonus of making the job of staff more rewarding and less stressful.

STAFF TRAINING

A significant area of stress for staff is anxiety about whether they have the appropriate training for the job they are doing.

The training of almost all health professionals is singularly lacking in any development of interpersonal skills. Recently at least one British hospital has begun to include this in its medical training programme, taking the subject seriously enough to employ actors to role play situations with doctors. This is very much an exception. Generally doctors are expected to acquire a 'bedside manner' through the discredited industrial practice of 'sitting by Nellie'.

Nurses, ultrasonographers and other health professionals may have an afternoon's training in counselling skills or perhaps an optional course of a few days, but otherwise, they too learn – or not – on the job. Anxiety created by the absence of these skills is increased by the knowledge that for patients the most important aspects of an encounter with a health professional are the manner in which they are told things, the consideration they are shown and whether or not they feel able to express their emotions or to ask questions.

Even staff who have excellent skills may sometimes feel uncertain and uncomfortable about how they are handling a situation because they have no frame of reference. The British Association of Counselling offers guidelines for staff using counselling skills in their work (as distinct from staff working primarily as counsellors) and has produced a Code of Ethics and Practice (British Association of Counselling, 1989). This includes the suggestion that a user of counselling skills should have 'received sufficient training to be able to use them appropriately' and should maintain his/her level of competence. The code also suggests that while the user of counselling skills is responsible for their use within any existing code of ethics and practice governing their functional roles, he/she should be clear whose interests they are serving and that this may involve a discussion of any conflict of interests. It also looks at issues of confidentiality.

A great deal of the value of having some basic training in counselling skills is that the practitioner acquires a frame of reference for working with patients and an awareness of both his/her skills and their limitations. In addition to providing an understanding of the relationship, enhancing listening and communicating skills, training enables the practitioner to define the limits of what is on offer and to be clear when to refer elsewhere. Basic courses in counselling skills are offered by a variety of bodies. They are normally part-time, 2–4 hours a week, running for anything from 10–30 weeks. Information about courses may be obtained from the local education authority, from local colleges and universities, in London from Floodlight (a guide to adult education) and from the BAC Directory, *Training in Counselling and Psychotherapy*. Much shorter introductory courses can be run over one or two days, possibly in-house.

Most of the health professionals working in prenatal diagnosis who are using counselling skills are doing so in the context of a particular professional role, but there are those whose job is exclusively, or in a very large part, concerned with counselling parents. Some of these may be professionally trained counsellors; others may have evolved into the job. The British Association of Counselling Code of Ethics and Practice for Counsellors (British Association of Counselling, 1992) is quite clear that 'counsellors commit themselves to a basic training course in counselling and undertake further training at intervals'. Not only is a preliminary training essential but ongoing training, workshops, meetings, etc. are an important source of support and stimulation for professionals working in this taxing area.

STAFF SUPERVISION

The code also specifies that 'counsellors monitor their counselling work through regular supervision by professionally competent supervisors'. The competence required is in counselling and supervision. The supervisor's role is to help the counsellor look at the process of the counselling. He or she need not therefore have knowledge of genetics nor even necessarily of the health service, though this might be preferable.

Supervision protects both patients and counsellor and is an important source of support for someone who is often the only person in a department with an exclusive counselling role. Where there is unlikely to be funding for one-to-one supervision, it may be possible either to join or to create a group for supervision. At the least it should be possible to contact other professionals working in prenatal diagnosis and to meet together to discuss cases and support one another. It would be necessary to establish ground rules for confidentiality and the structure of the meetings.

While it is considered essential for full-time counsellors to have supervision, the code of practice for using counselling skills does not require that practitioners have supervision. However, regular formal meetings to discuss cases and general issues of patient management are a valuable source of support for staff. Such meetings may be departmentally-based, multidisciplinary or restricted to a particular professional group. The group can be chaired from within the group or have an outside facilitator.

SELF-HELP

In addition to encouraging a caring workplace culture, providing training and group support, it is important that managers encourage staff to take responsibility for managing their own stress. This includes encouraging staff to take their holiday entitlement in regular breaks and ensuring that staff do not work excessively long hours (this includes resisting the temptation to ask midwives who live on site to fill in whenever there is a staff shortage).

Stress can be effectively managed by developing a balanced lifestyle (Hanson, 1986). This means paying attention to what we eat, avoiding junk food and increasing the consumption of fruit, vegetables and whole grain cereals. It is ironic that eating 'healthily' can be very difficult in many hospitals where the readily available snacks are high in fat and low in fibre. Together with a moderate consumption of alcohol and ideally no cigarettes this would give our bodies the best chance to resist stress.

A balanced lifestyle also means taking regular, pleasurable exercise – if it is not pleasurable we will not keep it up and smiling makes it more effective! Regular rhythmic exercise – cycling, swimming, jogging and walking – all help dispel stress. We also need to be able to relax passively. For some, a couple of hours in front of the television, listening to music or reading a book may achieve this. Others, however, become so tense that even when they are asleep they are not relaxed. Activities such as yoga, *tai ch'i*, Alexander technique, relaxation classes and deep massage all help to undo the tensions we have learnt to hold deep in our muscles.

We also need to express ourselves through some form of

creativity. Some people may feel all their creativity goes into their work but individuals who cope best with stress have activities outside work such as cooking, gardening, painting, photography, writing, playing an instrument, collecting stamps, bird-watching, or dancing. Some creative activities are solitary (most of us need some solitude somewhere in our lives), but many are social. Having a network of social contacts – family, friends, fellow enthusiasts – is the final important aspect of combating stress and caring for ourselves.

It is important for individuals to understand that providing a caring service for patients is achieved not through self-sacrifice and neglect of our own interests but by taking good care of ourselves and those for whom we are responsible. Recognizing the stresses of working in the field of prenatal diagnosis is the beginning of helping staff to work more effectively.

REFERENCES

British Association of Counselling (1989) *Code of Ethics and Practice for Counselling Skills*, British Association of Counselling, Rugby, Warwickshire.

British Association of Counselling (1992) *Code of Ethics and Practice for Counsellors*, British Association of Counselling, Rugby, Warwickshire.

Cooper, C., Cooper, R. and Eaker, L. (1988) *Living with Stress*, Penguin, Harmondsworth, Middlesex.

Hanson, P. (1988) *The Joy of Stress*, Pan Books, London.

Hingley, P. and Cooper, C. (1986) *Stress and the Nurse Manager*, John Wiley, Chichester.

Jenkins, R. (1992) Prevalence of mental illness in the workplace, in *Prevention of Mental Ill-Health at Work: A Conference*, (eds R. Jenkins and N. Coney), HMSO, London.

National Association for Staff Support (1992) *A Charter for Staff Support*, National Association for Staff Support, Woking, Surrey.

Wright, B. (1989) Critical incidents. *Nursing Times*, **85**(19).

Glossary

allele: one of two or more alternative forms of a gene.

alpha fetoprotein (AFP): a protein made by the fetus that is present in the serum of pregnant women and tends to be found in increased amounts if the fetus has a neural tube defect and in decreased amounts if the fetus has Down syndrome.

amniocentesis: withdrawal of a small amount of fluid from the amniotic sac round the developing fetus to enable chromosome, DNA or biochemical studies to be done.

anencephaly: a specific type of neural tube defect caused by the failure of the upper part of the neural tube to close. This leads to a failure of development of the skull and brain. This malformation is incompatible with extrauterine life of more than a few days.

anomaly scan: a detailed ultrasound scan done for the purpose of looking at the fetal anatomy to enable identification of fetal malformations. Such scans are done routinely at many antenatal clinics in the United Kingdom at about 19 weeks of pregnancy.

ascertainment: the identification of individuals or families to be included in a study. The method of ascertainment will affect the results of the study.

autosome: any chromosome other than a sex chromosome. Humans have 22 pairs of autosomes.

base pair: a pair of nucleotides (adenine–guanine, cytosine–thymine) in DNA. The order of the base pairs determines the sequence of the amino acids that are assembled to form a protein.

blastocyst: an early preimplantation stage of embryonic development in which the cells of the developing fetus and placenta are arranged in the form of a hollow ball.

CARE: the Scottish self-help group for parents who have had a termination of pregnancy because of a fetal abnormality.

carrier: an individual who does not manifest a condition but who carries a gene for it and can therefore pass this gene on to offspring who may, under certain circumstances, exhibit the condition.

chorionic villus sampling (CVS): the sampling of tissue from the developing placenta (chorionic villi) in order to do chromosome or DNA studies. The sample can be obtained transabdominally or transvaginally.

chorionicity: the status of twins with regard to the membranes surrounding them (the **chorion**). A shared chorionic membrane indicates monozygotic (identical) twins, while separate chorion leave the question open. Chorionicity can often be determined on ultrasound scan.

chromosome: a rod-shaped body made of DNA found in the nucleus of every cell in the body. Chromosomes carry the genes which determine the characteristics of an individual. Humans have 23 pairs of chromosomes in each cell – 22 pairs of autosomes and one pair of sex chromosomes.

concordance: this refers to two individuals (often twins) both having or both not having the same trait (often an abnormality).

cystic fibrosis: a disease of the mucous-secreting glands of the lungs, the pancreas, the mouth, the gastrointestinal tract and the sweat glands. In the caucasian population, it is the commonest serious disease inherited in an autosomal recessive manner. If both parents are unaffected carriers of the disorder, on average one in four of their children will be affected.

cytogenetics: the science of examining chromosomes.

delta F508: the name given to the commonest mutation causing cystic fibrosis. In the United Kingdom it accounts for about 75% of mutations of the cystic fibrosis gene.

diagnostic test: a test which aims to determine with a very high degree of accuracy whether or not an individual has a particular disorder. This is regarded as the 'gold standard' test in a screening programme.

discordance: this refers to the situation where two individuals (often twins) are different in respect to a particular trait (for example one has the disorder and the other does not).

dizygous: describes twins arising from the fertilization of two different eggs. Genetically such twins are no more alike than any other sibling pair.

DNA: deoxyribonucleic acid – the material of which genes are composed.

dominant inheritance: the mode of inheritance that is character-ized by an individual manifesting a trait for which only one of the relevant pair of genes codes. If a condition is inherited dominantly, it can be passed on from an affected parent to an offspring, even though the other parent does not carry the gene for the disease. An affected parent will pass it on (on average) to half his or her children.

Down syndrome (trisomy 21): individuals with Down syndrome have an extra copy of chromosome 21 in each cell. They have varying degrees of mental handicap, a characteristic appearance and often some congenital malformations. It is the commonest single chromosome abnormality in liveborn children. The inci-dence increases with maternal age.

Duchenne muscular dystrophy: a disease causing severe pro-gressive muscle weakness and eventual death in affected boys. It is an X-linked disease (carried on the X chromosome). Carrier women are unaffected but on average half of their sons are affected and half of their daughters are unaffected carriers.

Edwards syndrome (trisomy 18): individuals with Edwards syn-drome have an extra copy of chromosome 18 in each cell. They usually have lethal congenital malformations so very few of them survive past infancy, but those few who do are severely mentally handicapped.

eugenics: this refers to attempts to 'improve' a species either through controlling who does and who does not reproduce or through controlling which of their genes are passed on and which are not. There is considerable debate (with understandable public concern) as to whether prenatal diagnosis with termination of affected fetuses and screening for carrier status is an attempt at eugenic control.

familial: 'running in families'.

fetal blood sampling: the withdrawal of a small amount of fetal blood (usually from the point where the umbilical cord inserts into the placenta) in order to do chromosome, DNA or biochemi-cal tests on it.

gamete: a reproductive cell (ovum or sperm).

gene: the biological unit of heredity. Genes are arranged along chromosomes in the nucleus of each cell. They are made up of DNA.

genetic markers: normal variations which occur between the chromosomes of different individuals allowing the identification of the source of a specific part of a particular chromosome (for example, which of the mother's two X chromosomes the fetus has inherited).

genotype: the genetic constitution of an organism. The total of all the genes carried by that person, whether expressed or not.

haemoglobinopathy: any disease of the blood associated with the presence of an abnormal haemoglobin in the red blood cells. The commonest such diseases are sickle cell anaemia (found most commonly in those of Afro-Caribbean origin) and thalassaemia (more prevalent in those of Middle Eastern, Mediterranean and Far Eastern origin). These diseases are inherited in an autosomal recessive manner so that, if both parents are unaffected carriers of the gene in question, on average one in four of their children will be affected.

haemophilia: a clotting disorder which causes sufferers to bleed easily. It is a genetic defect and the gene causing it is located on the X chromosome. Carrier women are not affected, but on average half of their sons will be affected and half of their daughters will be carriers.

heterozygous: carrying two different alleles (versions of the gene) for a particular trait. Unaffected carriers of recessively inherited disorders are heterozygous, as they have one faulty and one normal allele of the gene for that disease state. Individuals with dominant disorders are usually heterozygous and carry one normal allele and one faulty allele for the trait.

homozygous: carrying two identical alleles (versions of the gene) for a particular trait. Genetic traits which are recessive in character, such as blood group type O, are only manifested when an individual is homozygous for that trait.

human chorionic gonadotrophin: a hormone produced by the placenta that is found in the mother's serum. It tends to be present in increased amounts if the fetus has Down syndrome and in decreased amounts if the fetus has Edwards syndrome.

Huntington's disease: a late-onset progressive disease characterized by involuntary movements, dementia and eventual death. It is inherited as an autosomal dominant. An affected parent will (on average) pass it on to half his/her children. Because it is a late-onset disease, symptoms are unlikely to occur before the affected person has had children.

hypoplasia: underdevelopment.

iatrogenic disease: disease caused by medical investigations or treatments.

inversion: the turning around of a part of a chromosome. If no genetic material is gained or lost, the individual should not be affected.

karyotype: an individual's full chromosome complement.

linkage: genes which are located close to each other on the same chromosome tend to be transmitted together so that an individual who inherits one of them is likely to have inherited the other. This is known as **linkage**.

marker chromosome: a small extra chromosome fragment.

meiosis: the cell division which results in the daughter cells having only one chromosome from each chromosome pair. This is the mechanism by which egg and sperm cells are made.

metaphase: A stage of cell division during which the chromosomes are visible under a microscope and can be examined.

mitosis: the cell division which results in the daughter cells having the same chromosome complement as the original cell. This is the mechanism by which all cells other than egg and sperm cells are made.

monozygous: describes twins resulting from a split early on in embryonic development so that two individuals develop from one fertilized egg. Such twins are genetically identical.

mosaicism: the presence in one individual of two cell lines. One line may be normal and the other abnormal. This can be the result of one abnormal cell division early in embryonic development. The affect on the individual will depend on the ratio of abnormal to normal cells and the distribution of abnormal cells in the body.

mutation: a change in the gene resulting from an error made when the gene is being copied. It may result in altered gene function which could render the gene less effective, useless or harmful.

negative result: on a diagnostic test, this means that nothing abnormal has been found (i.e. a normal result). On a screening test, this means that the individual screened has been found to be in the low-risk category and not to require diagnostic testing.

neural tube defect: a failure of the neural tube to close at the appropriate time in embryonic development. The main types of neural tube defects are anencephaly, encephalocoele and spina bifida.

oestrogen: a hormone secreted by the ovaries and the placenta.

Patau syndrome (trisomy 13): individuals with Patau syndrome have an extra copy of chromosome 13 in each cell. They usually have lethal congenital malformations and so are unlikely to survive past early infancy. If they do survive they are severely mentally handicapped.

perinatal: occurring in or concerned with the time just before, during and after birth.

phenotype: the observable properties of an individual produced by the interaction between all his/her genes and the environment.

phenylketonuria: a severe, inherited metabolic disorder leading to mental deficiency. It is due to the inability of the individual to metabolize the amino acid phenylalanine. If it is diagnosed by a simple blood test soon after birth and the infant has a diet low in phenylalanine, mental handicap can be avoided to a large extent. It is inherited in an autosomal recessive manner so that if both parents carry the gene, on average one in four of their children will be affected.

polar body: the body containing the discarded set of chromosomes resulting from the meiotic division which produced the egg. Thus, those chromosomes found in the polar body will not be in the egg.

polyhydramnios: an excess of fluid in the amniotic sac.

positive result: on a diagnostic test this means that an abnormality has been found. On a screening test, this means that the individual has been found to be in the high-risk group and that a diagnostic test will be offered.

predictive value: the chance that a person found to be positive on a particular screening test does actually have the condition being screened for.

prenatal exclusion test: a test that cannot confirm that a fetus has a condition but can confirm that it definitely does not. It is used in Huntington disease. The test involves ascertaining whether or not the fetus inherited the chromosome which carries the relevant gene from the affected grandparent. If the fetus did not, then it could not have inherited the disease. If it did, there is a 50% chance that it inherited the faulty copy of the gene.

prevalence: the proportion of individuals in a population who have the condition in question at a specified time.

prior risk: this is the risk that an individual is thought to have for developing a particular condition, or having a baby with a particular condition, before further tests are done or before more information becomes available. The prior risk may then be altered in the light of new information.

progesterone: a hormone secreted by the corpus luteum in the ovary which prepares and maintains the uterus for pregnancy.

recessive inheritance: the mode of inheritance in which a condition is only manifest if both copies of the relevant gene code for that condition. An individual can only be affected with a recessively inherited disorder if both parents carry a gene for the disorder and both of them pass that gene on to the individual. When both partners are unaffected carriers of a recessively inherited disorder, on average one in four of their children will be affected with the disorder.

SATFA (Support Around Termination For Abnormality): A self-help group in England for parents who have had a termination of pregnancy because of fetal abnormality.

screening test: a test designed to identify those individuals who are at a high enough risk of having a particular disorder to warrant being offered a diagnostic test. A screening test may be an actual test, such as a blood test, or it may be just the asking of a question, such as 'How old are you?'.

sensitivity: the proportion of people actually affected with a condition who will be found to be positive on a screening test for that condition. It determines the false negative rate.

serum screening: a screening test which uses serum (blood without the blood cells or clotting factors). In pregnancy, tests done on the mother's serum can give clues about the condition of the fetus. Serum screening can now be done to check the likelihood that the fetus has Down syndrome or spina bifida.

sex linked disorder: a disorder which is carried on a sex chromosome. Usually such disorders are carried on the X chromosome, and typically they are manifested only by males since males have only one copy of the X chromosome. They are carried by females who because of the healthy copy of the gene found on their other X chromosome are not themselves affected.

sickle cell disease: a recessively inherited severe anaemia found most commonly in people of Afro-Caribbean origin. If both parents are unaffected carriers of the disorder, on average one in four of their children will be affected.

specificity: the proportion of people not affected by a disorder who will be found to be negative on a screening test for that disorder. It determines the false positive rate.

spina bifida: a failure of the neural tube to close at the appropriate time during embryonic development, resulting in defective development of the spine and spinal cord. This usually means that neural tissue is damaged and the result is at least partial paralysis below the lesion. It sometimes results in hydrocephaly.

superovulation: the maturation of many eggs during one menstrual cycle. This is artificially induced in preparation for *in vitro* fertilization.

syndrome: a recognized pattern of signs, symptoms or malformations.

Tay–Sachs disease: an inborn error of metabolism that is inherited in an autosomal recessive manner so that, if both parents carry the gene, on average one in four of their children will be affected. Affected individuals suffer from progressive muscular weakness, paralysis, mental deterioration, blindness and eventual death. It is a disease which mainly affects those of Ashkenazy Jewish origin.

teratogen: a chemical, virus, toxin or environmental factor (such as radiation or heat) which causes exposed fetuses to have congenital abnormalities.

thalassaemia: a form of severe anaemia which is inherited as an autosomal recessive condition. If both parents are unaffected carriers of the disorder, on average one in four of their children will be affected. There are different types of thalassaemia and they vary in severity. It is prevalent in people of Mediterranean, Middle Eastern and Far Eastern origin.

toxoplasmosis: a disease caused by infection with the parasite *Toxoplasma gondii*. A pregnant woman who contracts the illness may not have any symptoms, but it may cause severe neurological damage in an exposed fetus.

translocation: a rearrangement of chromosome material; either parts of two chromosomes have broken off and swapped places or two whole chromosomes are stuck together. If no genetic material is gained or lost, the translocation is balanced and should not cause any problems to the individual. However, the carrier of a balanced translocation is at risk of having children with an unbalanced translocation in which there is some extra or missing genetic material. Such an individual might suffer from severe physical or developmental handicap.

trisomy: the presence in each cell of three copies of a chromosome instead of a normal pair. In humans, most autosomal trisomies cause spontaneous abortion of the embryo, but trisomies of chromosome 13, 18 and 21 are seen in live births and result in serious handicap. Trisomies of the sex chromosomes have less serious consequences.

trisomy 13: *see* **Patau syndrome**

trisomy 18: *see* **Edwards syndrome**

trisomy 21: *see* **Down syndrome**

ultrasound scan: a visual image produced by bouncing low-energy ultrasound waves off an object. It is used for visualizing the fetus *in utero*.

Useful addresses in the United Kingdom

ACT (Action for the Care of families whose Children have life-threatening and Terminal Conditions)
The Institute of Child Health
Royal Hospital for Sick Children
St Michael's Hill
Bristol BS2 8BJ
Telephone 0272 221556

The British Association of Counselling
1 Regent Place
Rugby
Warwickshire CV21 2PJ

CARE
36 Canmore Place
Stewarton
Ayrshire KA3 5PS

Contact A Family (support group for families who care for children with special needs)
16 Sutton Ground
London SW1P 2HP
Telephone 071 222 2695

Foundation for the Study of Infant Deaths (FSID)
35 Belgrave Square
London SW1X 8QB
Telephone 071 235 1721 (24-hour help line)
071 235 0965 (general enquiries)

Genetic Interest Group (GIG) (an umbrella group of voluntary organizations concerned with genetic disorders – can supply addresses of support groups for specific genetic disorders)

Institute of Molecular Medicine
John Radcliffe Hospital
Oxford OX3 9DW
Telephone 0865 744002 (help line)
Fax 0865 222501

The Miscarriage Association (MA)
c/o Clayton Hospital
Northgate
Wakefield
West Yorkshire WSF1 3JS
Telephone 0924 200799
Answerphone 0924 830515

National Association for Staff Support (NASS)
Central Office
9 Caradon Close
Woking
Surrey GU21 3DU

The Stillbirth and Neonatal Death Society (SANDS)
28 Portland Place
London W1N 4DE
Telephone 071 436 5881 (help line)
071 436 7940 (administration and publications)

Support Around Termination For Abnormality (SATFA)
29-30 Soho Square
London W1V 6JB
Telephone 071 439 6124 (help line)
071 287 3753 (administration)

TAMBA (The Twins and Multiple Births Association)
PO Box 30
Little Sutton
South Wirral
L66 1TH
Telephone 051 348 0020

Index

45X syndrome, *see* Turner syndrome

AFP, *see* Serum screening
Abnormality, *see* Congenital
    abnormality
Abortion, *see* Termination
Alpha fetoprotein screening, *see*
    Serum screening
Amniocentesis
    anxiety 39–46
    compared to CVS 39–46
    conditions picked up by 57, 86–9,
        91–3
    counselling before 66, 75–8
    in multiple pregnancy 149
    risks 66, 71, 123
    terminations after 96
    why women have amniocentesis
        160
    see also prenatal diagnosis
Anencephaly, *see* Neural tube
    defects
Antenatal diagnosis, *see* Prenatal
    diagnosis
Audit 66, 67, 198

Bart's testing, *see* Serum screening
Bereavement
    counselling 152, 154, 159, 179–80,
        183, 196–7, 198–201
    management 166, 186
Biopsy, egg and embryo 118
Birth plans 136
Blood disorders, *see* Sickle cell
    anaemia; Thalassaemia
Blood sampling
    maternal, *see* Serum screening
    fetal, *see* Fetal blood sampling
Body language
    carer's 74, 111
    client's 82–3

CVS, *see* Chorionic villus sampling

Carers
    effects of prenatal diagnosis on
        146–7, 161, 166, 198, 202–11
    support 203
Carrier testing 59, 60
Case studies 80–83
    after late prenatal diagnosis
        139–46
Children
    parental feeling towards other
        children after termination 190
Choice, *see* Decision making
Chorionic villus sampling (CVS) 89,
    93, 96
    and anxiety 39–46
    miscarriage after 42
    outcome 42
    termination following 163
    see also prenatal diagnosis
Chorionicity 150
Chromosome abnormalities 86–93
    marker 92
    see also individual conditions
Communication skills 20, 71, 78,
    82–3, 100, 106, 109–15, 147
    men and communication skills
        177, 178
    giving information 70–85, 197
Confidentiality 4, 16–17
Conflict, dealing with 19–21
Congenital abnormality
    assessment of 64
    diagnosis 90, 92, 95, 157, 161
    late diagnosis of 133, 136–8
    prevalence 55
    in twins 149
Consent, informed
    to amniocentesis 72, 73
    ethical aspects 18
    legal aspects 28
    necessity for 71–2
    what constitutes 72–4, 77
Conscientious objection 206
Coping response 101–2

Cost benefit analysis 56, 66
Cost effectiveness analysis 56, 66
Counselling 70–84, 98–103, 192–8
  in ante natal clinic 75–7
  for carers 208
  ethical aspects 18–19
  information giving 72, 73, 86, 89,
    92, 93, 95, 137
  and *in vitro* fertilization 127
  justification for 70–72
  leaflets 78
  legal aspects 28
  non directive 18, 74–6, 98, 99
  after termination 169, 179
  what women want from 79–80
Counsellors
  code of practice 209
  see also carers
Cultural aspects of pregnancy loss
    xii, 97, 183
Cystic fibrosis 184
  carrier testing 59, 60
  preimplantation diagnosis 121,
    125
  in twins 150, 153

DMD, *see* Duchenne muscular
    dystrophy
Decision making
  counselling 73–4
  decision tree 101–2
  after late prenatal diagnosis 135,
    138
  living with the choice 195–8
  models 61, 99–102
  pressures on 164, 185, 193–4
  psychological factors 97, 99–101,
    103
  about termination 94–9, 165
  value of 50, 157, 159, 162, 163
  see also counselling
Deontological approach to ethics 7,
    13
Diabetes 55, 59
Diagnostic tests, *see* Amniocentesis;
    Chorionic villus sampling
Dizygosity 150, 151
Doctor–patient relationship 15–17
Down syndrome 86, 158, 162, 163
  case studies 81, 82
  counselling 76–8
  duty to treat 34
  and maternal age 57, 66, 67

in preimplantation diagnosis 122
in twins 149, 150, 153
see also serum screening
Duchenne muscular dystrophy
    (DMD) 93–5, 96, 120, 121, 150,
    160
Duty to treat 34

Edwards syndrome (trisomy 18) 86
  case studies 139–42, 144–6
Embryo transfer 118
Emotional reactions 158–70
  of carers to late termination 146,
    182
  determinants of 170, 184, 187,
    198
  of father 173–80, 188, 189, 198
  guilt 164
  loss of self esteem 192
  of parents to late diagnosis 137,
    138
  to selective fetocide 151–5
  after subsequent baby 195
  to termination 123, 181–98
Epidemiology 55, 56
Epidermolysis bullosa 150
Ethical issues 1–21, 97, 100, 102,
    191–2, 195
  preimplantation diagnosis 129
  selective fetocide 151
  status of fetus 11–15
Eugenics 61, 151

FBS, *see* Fetal blood sampling
False negative 57
  in amniocentesis 77
False positive 57, 58, 67
Family
  structure 96
  support from 190, 191
Fetal blood sampling (FBS) 93
Fetal sexing 32, 33, 94, 121
Fetal viability 33, 134
Fetocide
  bereavement 152–4
  complications 151
  emotional reactions of carers to
    154–5
  emotional reaction of parents to
    151–5
  emotional reactions of survivors
    154–5
  ethical issues 151

Fetocide *contd*
  indications 150
  methods 145, 150
  risks 151
  selective 149–55
  selective reduction 152
  side effects 151
  in survivor of multiple
    pregnancy 152, 153, 154, 159,
    164, 165, 169
Fetus
  in different cultures 183
  status of 1–15
Fragile X 125
Friends, support from 190, 191

GP, *see* Primary care
General practitioner (GP), *see*
    Primary care
Genetic screening, *see* Screening
    programmes
Gestational age, at termination 96,
    163
Grief
  of father 175, 176, 177, 182–3
  after subsequent baby 182, 195
  of survivor of multiple
    pregnancy 152, 153, 154, 159,
    164, 165, 169
Guilt 155, 164, 169, 175, 194

Handicap
  intellectual 84, 88, 90–92
Haemoglobinopathies, *see* Sickle
    cell anaemia; Thalassaemia
Haemophilia 120
  in twins 150, 153
High risk groups 38, 55, 57, 59, 93
Higher order pregnancies, *see*
    Multiple pregnancy
Human Fertilization and
    Embryology Act 32–3, 130,
    134, 138
Huntington's disease 94, 102
Hurler syndrome 150

IVF, *see* In vitro fertilization
Iatrogenic disease 62
In vitro fertilization (IVF) 29, 117,
    118, 123–9
  case study 81
Infanticide 138
Infertility 87–90, 95, 97

Informed consent, *see* Consent
Insurance 60
Inversion 91

Klinefelter syndrome (XXY
    syndrome) 77, 86, 87, 90, 97
  in twins 150

Language delay 87–8, 91
Legal aspects 20–35
  and preimplantation diagnosis
    129
Lesch–Nyhan syndrome 120
Linkage analysis 94
Listening
  the importance of 82–83
  see also communication skills

Marital relationship 189–90
Malformation, *see* Congenital
    abnormality
Maternal age
  and prenatal screening 45, 49,
    126, 198
Microcephaly
  in twins 150
Miscarriage
  after chorionic villus sampling
    and amniocentesis 42
Monosomy, *see* Turner syndrome
Monozygosity 150, 151
Moral frameworks 11
Mosaicism 86, 90, 92, 93, 95
Multiple pregnancy 149–55
  congenital malformations 149
  chorionicity 150
  dichorionicity 150
  higher order 152
  and *in vitro* fertilization 125
  monochorionicity 150
  surviving twin 154, 155
  ultra sound scanning in 110
Muscular dystrophy, *see* Duchenne
    muscular dystrophy

National Health Service (NHS) and
    prenatal diagnosis
  legal aspects 25–35, 63
NTD, *see* Neural tube defects
Neural tube defects
  case study on anencephaly 80
  in twins 149, 150, 153, 175

and randomized controlled trials 182
and screening 184
Nightmares 188
Non directive counselling, *see* Counselling

Ovum donation 89

Parents
   age 96–7
   autonomy 99
   expectations 90, 97–8
Patau syndrome (trisomy 13) 86
Philosophical approach 5–10
Photographs 176
Post mortems 153, 166, 167
Predective testing 94
Predictive value 58
Preimplantation diagnosis 116–32
Prenatal diagnosis
   definition 1
   effects on parents 163
   late diagnosis 134–47
   legal aspects 29–31
   and maternal age 45, 126, 198
   see also chorionic villus sampling; amniocentesis; fetal blood sampling; preimplantation diagnosis
Prenatal exclusion test 94
Prevalence 58, 59
Primary care 55
Prior risk 73
Professional staff, *see* Carers
Prospective new born studies 87–90
Psychological factors, *see* Decision making 97, 102
Public health 56, 57, 59, 67
   definition 54
Public policy on screening 25, 63, 67

Quality of life, 2, 3
   of child 71, 162
   mother and rest of family 162, 163, 206

Randomized controlled trials 64
   amniocentesis and chorionic villus sampling 41–2
   preconception vitamin supplementation 182
   ultrasound 64

Recessive disorders 59, 60
   and preimplantation diagnosis 120, 125
   see also individual conditions
Religious beliefs 97
   case study 80
Religious support 136, 140
Renal malformations
   case study 142–3
Reproductive conflict 193, 194
Resources 24, 25, 56, 63, 65, 67, 131, 157, 167
Risks, *see* High risk groups 100, 102
Rubella 55, 64

SATFA, *see* Support Around Termination For Abnormality; Support groups
Screening 54–67
   cut offs 38
   definition 57
   false negatives 38, 57
   false positives 38, 57
   predictive value 58
   sensitivity 58
   specificity 58
   see also screening programmes
Screening programmes 57
   anxiety 37, 43–6
   carrier testing 60
   criteria for success 62
   Down syndrome, *see* Serum screening
   objectives 61
   research and development 66
   sensitivity 58
   specificity 58
   toxoplasmosis 65
   uptake of 59, 60, 67, 135, 137
   see also serum screening
Selective fetocide, *see* Fetocide
Self fulfilling prophecy 91
Self help groups, *see* Support groups; Useful addresses
   general 196
   SATFA 158–70, 173–80
Sensitivity 58
Serum screening for Down syndrome 66, 67, 76, 184, 187
   and anxiety 39–46
   public health aspects 66
   women's experience of 43–9
Sex, *see* Fetal sexing

Sex chromosome abnormality 89
Sex linked, *see* X linked
Sexual problems following
    termination 189, 190
Sickle cell anaemia 60, 75, 120, 121
Social pressures 98, 100
Socioeconomic factors 97, 102
Specificity 58
Spina bifida, *see* Neural tube defects
Staff, *see* Carers
Stillbirth 136
Stress
    for carers 202–9
    causes 202–3
    coping with 205–6
    dealing with, for carers 207, 208,
        212
    effects on carers 204
    ideal amount 205
    associated with prenatal
        diagnosis 206
Structural chromosome
    rearrangements, *see*
    Translocations
Supernumary marker
    chromosomes 92
Supervision
    of staff 210–11
Support Around Termination For
    Abnormality (SATFA) 167,
    168, 173
Support groups
    patient 136, 177, 179–80, 203
    carers 211
    useful addresses 222–3

Tay–Sachs disease 57, 75, 120, 121,
    150
Tentative pregnancy 41, 161
Teratogens 55, 93
Termination of pregnancy
    following amniocentesis 96
    effects on carers 147, 148
    effects on parents 163–71, 173–80,
        185–98
    ethical approaches 13–21, 191
    factors affecting decision
        regarding 90, 94–9, 101
    late 134–47
    legal aspects 32–5
    management 136, 163, 165, 196–8

public health issues and 60, 65
support after 167, 175–6, 180, 186
see also fetocide
Thalassaemia 57, 150
Thalidomide 55
Toxoplasmosis screening 65–6
Training
    of carers 107, 209–10
Translocation 86, 91, 95, 120
Triple testing, *see* Serum screening
Triple X syndrome 86, 87, 90, 98
Trisomy 21, *see* Down syndrome
Trisomy 18, *see* Edwards syndrome
Trisomy 13, *see* Patau syndrome
Tuberculosis 67
Turner syndrome 89, 90, 120
    in twins 150
Twins, *see* Multiple pregnancy

Ultrasound screening 76, 106–15
    as aid to bonding 183
    and decision to terminate 90–93,
        96
    as diagnostic test 72, 73
    effectiveness 64, 72
    evaluation of 64
    late in pregnancy 137
    as memento of dead fetus 154
    public health aspects of 64
    women's experience 46–8, 96,
        137, 140
Utilitarian approach 7, 13, 56
Utilities 101

Written information 73, 77
Worst case scenarios 74, 101
Wrongful life claims 31

X linked conditions 120
    mental retardation 94
    and preimplantation diagnosis
        125
    see also Duchenne muscular
        dystrophy; fragile X;
        haemophilia; Lesch–Nyhan
        syndrome
XXX syndrome, *see* Triple X
    syndrome
XXY syndrome, *see* Klinefelter
    syndrome
XYY syndrome 88, 98